10-Minute Balance Exercises for Seniors

Fully Illustrated Home Workout Guide with 58 Simple Exercises to Improve Stability, Core Strength, Prevent Falls & Gain Independence - Video Included!

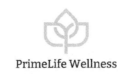

PrimeLife Wellness

Published by: PrimeLife Wellness

Visit our website at primelife-wellness.com.

Contact us at team@primelife-wellness.com.

Ebook ISBN: 978-1-915710-50-5

Paperback ISBN: 978-1-915710-51-2

Hardcover ISBN: 978-1-915710-52-9

CONTENTS

FOREWORD BY MATHIEU SONIER

As a healthcare professional, I've witnessed the impact of effective balance exercises that I regularly prescribe to my patients. One particular memory comes to mind: an older woman, previously limited by her fear of falling, now confidently engages in all the everyday activities she loves after diligently practicing these exercises. Moments like these attest to the transformative power of balance-focused interventions.

From my first encounter with James at PrimeLife Wellness, I felt his deep commitment to the well-being of others, a sentiment that resonates within me. Our shared passion for the importance of exercise in the older population has driven me to collaborate with him on this book. James' commitment to helping others is felt within these pages.

This book stands out for its clear explanation of why balance is essential at every age. It highlights the often-overlooked importance of balance and its significant impact on life quality, especially for older adults. The selection of exercises in this book has been well-curated, addressing all aspects of balance. You will also find two well-designed 30-day programs that fit your needs, starting your journey toward a more balanced life.

In collaborating with PrimeLife Wellness, our goal is to produce a resource that not only provides exercises but also explores the reasons behind the importance of balance. We invite you to join us in discovering why balance is crucial, not only as a preventive strategy but also as a key element of a fulfilling life. This book reflects our joint commitment to caring for seniors and emphasizes the need to prioritize balance in their lives.

Mathieu Sonier

Licensed Clinical Physiotherapist

Montreal, Canada

HOW TO ACCESS THE VIDEO DEMONSTRATIONS

Welcome to 10-Minute Balance Exercises for Seniors! With this book comes complete video demonstrations of every exercise and balance test. These videos provide clear, visual demonstrations, ensuring you perform the exercises safely and effectively.

To Access the Demonstrations:

1. Retrieve the passcode at the end of this book.

2. Visit our website, PrimeLife-Wellness.com, and click on 'Video Demonstrations.'

3. Enter the passcode.

Also on Our Website:

1. **PDF Copy of the Workout Tracker:** At the end of this book, you'll find two 30-day workout plans followed by a blank tracker to record your progress. We've also provided a downloadable PDF version of this tracker on our website, allowing you to reuse it as needed.

2. **Email Community Subscription:** Join our email

community to get the following benefits sent straight to your inbox:

- Be part of our advanced review team and get future books for free.

- Optimizing nutrition for senior fitness success ebook.

- Breathing techniques to enhance your workout's effectiveness ebook.

Access these resources by visiting our website. Type the URL into your browser or scan the QR code below with your phone.

PrimeLife-Wellness.com

INTRODUCTION

*"Those who think they have no time for bodily
exercise will sooner or later have to find time for
illness." - Edward Stanley*

You open the car door and step out. You feel the hot sun beating down on you. Quickly, you put on a wide-brimmed hat to shield your neck, so harshly exposed to the scorching sunlight. A few quick paces, and you're at the trunk, not wasting any time as the moisture from your body is sucked through the pores in your skin. Deck chair strap on your shoulder, umbrella in hand, cooler in the other, trunk closed, car locked. Grandchildren in tow, you look ahead through your sunglass lenses at the undulating sand dunes between you and your beach oasis.

You feel a bead of sweat drip down your face. Is it from the heat? Or is there a hint of apprehension about the challenging walk ahead, the uneven terrain that could test your balance? This worry isn't uncommon. For many seniors, the fear of falling is a constant companion, shadowing every step. Falls are not just physical setbacks; they become barriers to independence, eroding the confidence we once had in our bodies. While a natural process, aging can diminish our reaction times and physical strength, making even a walk across sand dunes feel like an odyssey. The anxiety of a potential fall can turn joyful moments into sources of stress, limiting our world more than we'd like to admit.

But imagine a different scenario. What if dedicating just a small portion of your day to balance exercises could transform these moments of apprehension into ones of confidence and independence? Envision being able to traverse the sand dunes with ease, the fear of falling replaced by reassuring certainty in every step. This is not a far-fetched dream, and research confirms it.

A British Journal of Sports Medicine study found that in a sample of 12,981 people aged 60 or over, regular exercise reduced the rate of falls by 23%, increasing to 24% when the participants specifically did balance and functional exercises. If the participant did multiple forms of exercise, most commonly balance exercises mixed with strength or resistance training, that number rose to 34%. Just 10 minutes of such exercises each day could be the key to maintaining your independence and enjoying life's simple pleasures, like a day at the beach with your grandchildren, without fear.

Our easy-to-follow guide makes the path to this newfound confidence and independence clear and attainable. The first step is understanding what balance truly is–the mechanics behind it, its vital importance, especially as we age, and how it profoundly impacts our daily lives. To help you grasp where you currently stand, we'll guide you through simple methods to assess your own balance. This initial assessment is crucial, as it not only provides a starting point but also helps you track your progress as you move forward. Then, we will cover the exercises, each specifically tailored for seniors. You'll find exercises that suit your needs regardless of your fitness level or mobility. We'll guide you through various types, including:

- **Seated exercises** for those who need to start with a more gentle approach.

- **Standing routines** to build strength and stability.

- **Walking drills** that enhance coordination and endurance.

- **Floor-based movements** focusing on mobility and overall balance.

- **Core exercises** to improve your body's ability to not get injured.

- **Vestibular exercises** that specifically target the inner ear balance system.

If some of these terms are new to you, don't worry. Each exercise type is explained in detail, with step-by-step instructions on how to perform them safely and effectively. Adjustments and variations are provided so you can tailor the exercises to your capabilities. We conclude with two structured 30-day exercise plans designed to progressively improve your balance, strength, and confidence.

Each confident step across the sand dunes highlights the importance of balance. This guide is your key to transforming worry into certainty, enabling you to navigate life's uneven terrains easily. Imagine moving across the dunes with your grandchildren, each step steady and secure, thanks to the simple exercises you've incorporated into your daily routine.

Who is PrimeLife Wellness?

Hello, I'm James Evans, the lead author and driving force behind PrimeLife Wellness. Our mission is to empower seniors with the tools they need for a healthier, more independent life. Recognizing a significant gap in accessible, effective balance exercises for seniors, we sought to create a scientifically sound and easy-to-follow resource.

My journey into the world of fitness began as a competitive rower at university. This experience instilled in me a deep appreciation for physical fitness and its impact on quality of life. In 2020, while surfing in Australia, I slipped a disc in my spine. The surgeon advised me that it might not heal naturally and invasive spinal surgery could be a necessity. This marked the beginning of a two-year journey of physiotherapy, personal training, and Pilates. A long recovery followed, where I not only healed but also returned to fitness stronger than ever, now competing in CrossFit.

I collaborated with experienced physiotherapist Mathieu Sonier to develop this book. With over a decade of clinical experience at the time of writing, Mathieu's expertise was invaluable in curating the best exercises to improve your balance while ensuring a safe and effective route to greater independence. His diligence, experience, and passion for helping people with physiotherapy have really elevated this book.

My partner, a skilled Pilates instructor working with top-end clients in London, also played a crucial role in creating this book. Her insights into Pilates and its benefits for body alignment and core strength were vital. Together, along with a team of experienced researchers, we've crafted this book to address a significant gap in accessible and practical balance exercises for seniors.

At PrimeLife Wellness, we aim to empower seniors with the tools they need for a healthier, more independent life. This book is more than just a guide; it's an ally in your journey toward greater balance, confidence, and independence. Now, let's move on to the first chapter, where we'll delve into understanding what balance really is.

THE IMPORTANCE OF BALANCE

According to the CDC, "About 36 million falls are reported among seniors each year, resulting in more than 32,000 deaths." These astounding statistics would make pretty much anyone over a certain age pause. Most of these falls result from a lack of flexibility and balance. These falls are one of the most common reasons seniors can no longer live independently in their own homes. This shows how important cultivating and improving flexibility and balance can be to your safety and well-being.

Balance is one of those terms that is not necessarily easy to define. You certainly know what it is when you lack it, though. The CDC simplifies the idea of balance by discussing postural control. This means being able to hold, move into, or return to a specific body position. If our weight is unevenly spread, it can be hard to maintain postural control, leading to slips, falls, and potential injuries.

Many people get hurt from slips and falls due to bad balance, sometimes causing minor injuries like bruises but other times leading to serious harm like broken bones or concussions. It's important to distinguish these balance-related falls from those caused by other health issues, like seizures. For our discussion, we're focusing only on falls caused by loss of balance.

You might not think falling is as risky as it truly is, but the statistics are frightening. For people over the age of 65, falls were the 7th leading cause of death in 2018. That same year, some 3 million emergency room visits resulted from falls in people over 65. For many, these falls ultimately mean they must leave their homes and independence behind. There is even a trend where seniors fail to report falls they may have experienced as they are afraid it will result in them no longer being able to stay in their homes.

Types of Balance

For our discussion, we want to focus on two kinds of balance: static and dynamic.

Static Balance

This term refers to our ability to stay stationary and in one place. It is our ability to get in and stay in a specific posture, such as squatting. Think about standing on one leg. You aren't moving, but you must have your center of mass in the proper position to stay stable. If you are struggling with overall balance issues, this is likely where you will begin with your balance routine. You must have a decent amount of static balance before focusing on your dynamic balance.

Dynamic Balance

Dynamic balance involves maintaining stability as you move, such as walking without tripping or falling. This requires continuously shifting your weight and is generally more challenging than static balance, where you stay still. Strengthening your static balance before progressing to dynamic balance exercises is beneficial. Still, both forms are crucial for your safety and independence. In later sections of this guide, we will introduce specific exercises to enhance static and dynamic balance.

How Our Bodies Balance Themselves

Balance might seem like just shifting weight to stay stable, but it's actually more complex. It involves three main parts: our vision (seeing), proprioception (feeling), and the vestibular system (inner ear balance). These three work together to keep upright. Each one is important for good balance.

Visual System

Our eyes help us understand light and color, which is crucial for knowing where we are and keeping our balance. Inside our eyes, there are special cells called cones and rods. Cones let us see colors and clear images in bright light, while rods help us see in low light. These cells change what we see into signals that go to our brain, giving us important details about our surroundings. This information is not just for seeing but also helps us keep our balance.

Proprioceptive System

This system is vital to our body's understanding and interaction with the world. It involves sensors in our muscles, joints, and connective tissues that detect movement and pressure. These sensors send signals to the brain, much like our eyes do with visual information, allowing us to perceive the position and movement of our limbs and body. This system is essential for coordinating movements and maintaining balance.

Vestibular System

This system, primarily located in the inner ear, is crucial in maintaining balance and spatial orientation. It consists of specialized structures that detect head movements and changes in position. When we move our heads, this system sends signals to the brain, allowing us to understand our orientation in space. It is vital not only for balance and coordination but also for perceiving the direction of sounds.

What Changes With Age?

As we age, our sensory systems, like sight, hearing, and musculoskeletal functions, often weaken, impacting our balance and posture. Understanding these changes is crucial, even though we can't completely prevent them. Balance issues become more common with age because our brain receives less accurate sensory information. This is due to not just hearing and vision loss but also changes in our muscles and joints.

Dizziness is also a frequent issue for seniors and those with certain health conditions, further affecting balance. Balance disorders, medical conditions, or medications can cause this. While we can't eliminate these factors, understanding and adapting to them can improve our balance and safety at home. The interplay of these systems—muscle strength, joint flexibility, eyesight, and inner ear function—is vital for orientation and staying upright. Loss of muscle mass, joint stiffness, eye and ear problems, and medication side effects can all alter our brain's perception, affecting balance.

Limitations and Health Issues Affecting Balance

Now that we understand the three main systems that interact to help us balance and orient ourselves, let's look at how ailments or issues can impact our balance.

Medications and Balance

Harvard Medical School notes that while medications have their benefits, they can also lead to side effects like dizziness, impaired alertness, fatigue, and blurred vision, all of which can negatively impact our balance. These side effects are particularly relevant when considering the three sensory systems responsible for balance discussed earlier. The interaction of medications, especially in seniors who often take multiple prescriptions, can increase the risk of these adverse effects. For example, blood pressure medications, commonly used by seniors, frequently cause dizziness and lightheadedness.

Seniors should have their healthcare providers periodically review their medications. Over time, people tend to accumulate prescriptions, and a re-evaluation might reveal that some drugs are no longer necessary. Reducing the number of medications can often alleviate balance problems caused by their side effects.

Chronic Health Conditions

Balance issues can stem from various health conditions, with inner ear problems being among the most common. The inner ear's role in maintaining balance is often underestimated, and any impairment, such as hearing loss or damage, can disrupt these signals. Similarly, visual impairments also impact balance. While it's commonly understood that vision helps us orient ourselves, the inner ear's contribution to balance is equally, if not more, significant.

The National Institutes of Health identifies several other conditions that can lead to balance difficulties, including stroke, diabetes, thyroid issues, and heart disease. Gait abnormalities, which refer to how we walk, also play a critical role in balance and mobility. Factors such as foot problems, muscle or tendon disorders, and arthritis can alter our gait, making it more challenging to maintain balance and increasing the risk of falls.

Cognitive Health Issues

Cognitive issues can also affect mobility and balance in seniors. While occasional forgetfulness is normal with aging, severe memory loss can hinder self-care and movement. Conditions like Alzheimer's and dementia are well-known for causing mobility problems, but other cognitive issues can also impact a senior's ability to move around.

Mental health issues such as depression and anxiety can impact mobility and balance in seniors by reducing physical activity and exercise. Sleep disorders, common in older adults, can cause reduced alertness and mental clarity. This can negatively affect mobility, making it harder for the brain to process signals needed for balance and fall prevention.

Environmental Hazards

So far, we've discussed health issues affecting mobility in seniors, but environmental factors are also important. This includes anything in our surroundings, indoors or outdoors, that can affect safe movement. For example, stairs become a challenge as we age due to slower reflexes and stiffer muscles and joints, making it harder for seniors to navigate them safely.

Many home features, such as slippery rugs, clutter, and poor lighting, can increase the risk of tripping and falling. To reduce the risk of falls, it's helpful to examine your home and identify potential hazards that you can remove to make your living space safer.

Uneven terrain and poor landscaping are common outdoor hazards for seniors. For example, leaves left on the yard or sidewalk can become slippery when wet, increasing the risk of falls. If you cannot manage these tasks, having someone else clean up can significantly reduce the chance of falls.

Consequences of Poor Balance

There are a lot of problems that can come about as a result of poor balance. The most obvious are the physical injuries sustained when one trips and falls. But there are also psychological and social impacts.

Physical Consequences

Falls can cause injuries, from minor bruises and cuts to more serious ones, like broken bones. A broken bone can further reduce mobility and take longer to heal in older adults, potentially leading to a decline in overall health. Additionally, falls can result in head injuries, including concussions or traumatic brain injuries, which can have long-lasting health impacts beyond mobility issues. In some cases, injuries from falls may lead to long-term disability.

Psychological Impact

While physical injuries are a concern, the psychological effects are also significant. Fear of falling is common, and a certain level of fear can be helpful, making us more cautious. However, excessive fear can impact the quality of life. Fear may lead us to avoid certain places and activities, increasingly restricting our movement and experiences. This fear can cause significant psychological stress and trauma, especially for those who have experienced a fall. This anxiety can erode confidence and limit the willingness to engage in activities, reducing life's enjoyment and possibilities.

Economic and Social Impact

Poor balance and the risk of falls are not only physically harmful but also have significant economic impacts. The CDC reports that fall-related medical expenses are about $50 billion annually. This cost results from increasing healthcare prices and the additional care needed for seniors, who often take longer to heal. Long-term consequences like disability can lead to expenses for rehabilitation, medication, and home modifications.

There's also a social impact to consider. Those injured in falls may become more dependent on family members or medical professionals, creating stress and strain for caregivers and feelings of dependence in the injured person.

Importance of Preventing Falls

Preventing falls is crucial as it reduces safety risks and helps maintain independence in older age, leading to a fuller and better quality of life.

Safety

One effective way to lower the risk of trips and falls is through balance exercises. These exercises are crucial for enhancing physical well-being and safety. A research study in France found that participating in balance exercise programs can reduce the risk of bone fractures by 61%, significantly decreasing the likelihood of serious injury. This finding applies to regular seniors with common health issues, who experienced a notable reduction in fall risk through these exercises.

Independence

Falls and related injuries are a major reason seniors lose their ability to live independently at home. By improving balance, not only do you enhance your safety and reduce the risk of falls, but you also maintain your independence. Working on balance is an investment in your ability to stay autonomous and live life as you choose.

Quality of Life

People living in assisted care facilities or relying heavily on others often report a lower quality of life compared to those living independently. Having control over daily life is valuable, and this autonomy can be limited when dependent on others. By improving balance, you equip yourself to stay active, even as you age, helping maintain your independence and quality of life.

What Is the Solution?

Balance exercises are a great solution if you have poor balance and are unsure how to improve it. These exercises can significantly enhance your health and well-being, helping you stay independent and active. Engaging in balance exercises has many positive effects.

Strengthening Muscles

We discussed how muscle loss, joint stiffness, and similar issues from the three key systems can decrease balance and mobility. Evidence suggests that reduced strength contributes to seniors' higher fall risk. Balance exercises strengthen muscles, enhancing overall balance. A stronger core means the muscles providing upper body stability are more effective. They also boost stamina and endurance, and improve joint motion and posture.

Improved Stability

Recalling our discussion on static and dynamic balance, research indicates that core exercises focusing on balance can enhance body stability. This means a more stable spine supporting you in an upright, balanced position. Balance exercises improve weight distribution for stability and aid in dynamic balance. With improved stability, you'll find it easier to change positions without losing balance.

Enhancing Coordination

Coordination, crucial for moving safely without falling, is the smooth execution of physical movements. For those with balance issues, poor coordination is often a problem. Balance exercises can improve coordination. As you practice and gain control over fine movements, it becomes easier to coordinate different body parts to move as intended.

Building Confidence

We discussed how fear, especially of falling, can impact quality of life. Engaging in balance exercises builds body strength and skills, boosting confidence in our mobility. This increased confidence reduces fear and allows us to continue enjoying activities. As we age, our bodies change, leading to potential hearing and vision loss and health issues, which can affect mobility and balance. Improving balance is vital to maintaining independence and safety.

Enhancing balance can significantly improve quality of life in later years by increasing both physical strength and confidence. Now that we understand balance, its impact, and improvement methods, let's explore ways to test and assess balance.

HOW TO TEST YOUR BALANCE

For adults over 65, one-third have balance problems, which rises to over half for those over 75. This statistic highlights the importance of balance for maintaining independence, especially with age. Starting with balance tests helps us understand our current balance abilities, track progress, and determine where to modify exercises to make them easier or harder.

There are four main tests that we will discuss in this chapter:

- Romberg

- 5-Time Sit-to-Stand

- Functional Reach

- Timed Up & Go

These tests help assess your current level of balance and ability. Everyone has unique needs and limitations, so the later exercises are categorized into beginner, intermediate, and challenging levels. Your performance in these tests will indicate the most suitable starting point for your balance exercises. By knowing your starting point and following appropriate exercises, you can improve your balance and avoid becoming a part of the concerning statistics related to balance issues.

The Importance of Balance Tests

Balance tests are more than just diagnostic tools; they enhance overall safety. By pinpointing specific balance weaknesses, these tests can direct attention to environmental modifications that could prevent falls. For example, home modifications like adding railings or removing trip hazards can be considered if a test reveals difficulty moving around (like in the Timed Up & Go test.)

In addition to identifying physical challenges, these tests can be motivational. Seeing tangible improvements in balance over time can be encouraging and empowering. This psychological benefit is as important as the physical one, as it can lead to increased enthusiasm and commitment to maintaining regular exercise.

Balance Assessment Criteria

- **Posture** refers to maintaining proper alignment of the body, ensuring that the spine is correctly positioned and the body is balanced, whether sitting or standing.

- **Stability** refers to how well you can hold your position without shifting, swaying, or wobbling.

- **Coordination** refers to how smoothly you can move between positions without issues or struggles.

- **Recovery** refers to how quickly and easily you can right yourself when you get off balance.

- **Focus** refers to how well you can remain balanced while doing an unrelated activity (such as washing dishes.)

- **Adaptability** refers to how easily and effectively you can adjust your balance when necessary.

People's skills in these areas vary greatly. They may change over time, highlighting the usefulness of balance exercises for both initial assessment and ongoing monitoring.

How Does Testing My Balance Help Me Determine My Exercise Routine?

Knowing your current ability level is crucial before starting balance exercises; balance tests are an effective way to assess this. If your balance is good, you can start with more advanced exercises, while those with weaker balance should begin at a lower level.

Starting at the appropriate level is essential to avoid injury and discouragement. Attempting exercises that are too difficult can lead to frustration. It's better to start with more straightforward activities and realistically set achievable goals, allowing steady progress.

Balance tests evaluate different aspects of balance, helping identify specific areas needing improvement. For instance, you might need more focus on standing than sitting exercises. The results from these tests provide valuable information, enabling you to tailor your exercise routine effectively to your needs.

The Tests

Now, let's take a look at the four most common balance tests. It's essential to understand your limitations and ensure you have someone to help if you need it. Remember, you can find video demonstrations of all these tests on our website, PrimeLife-Wellness.com.

Ensure you have someone to help support should you fall off balance. Testing your balance alone, without someone to catch you, can be dangerous and should be avoided at all costs.

Romberg

The Romberg test involves standing with your feet together, and arms crossed over your chest, aiming to maintain this position steadily for one minute. If successful, the next step is to repeat with your eyes closed. For a more advanced test, stand with one foot in front of the other as if balancing on a narrow beam.

Failing the test means shifting your feet for balance or grabbing something for support.

If you struggle with the initial test, begin with basic seated balance exercises. If you complete all stages successfully, you can start with intermediate.

5-Time Sit-to-Stand

This test evaluates your ability to move from sitting to standing safely and smoothly, assessing balance, weight transfer, and leg strength.

To perform this test, you need a standard chair and a timer. Sit in the chair with your arms crossed, then stand up and sit down five times consecutively, ensuring you don't risk falling.

Start the timer as you begin the sequence. Ideally, you should complete this within 15 seconds. Taking longer indicates a higher fall risk, suggesting you should start with basic sitting exercises.

Functional Reach

This test evaluates your ability to maintain balance while reaching forward. For safety, do this with someone and near a countertop, where you can place a tape measure or ruler to measure your reach and grab for support if needed.

Stand with your feet slightly apart and extend your arm forward to set a starting point to measure from. Then, reach as far ahead as possible without losing balance, and measure the distance.

If you can only reach six inches or less in this test, it suggests a high risk of falling. In this case, you should concentrate on beginner and seated exercises. Reaching between six to ten inches indicates a moderate fall risk, so you should not begin with exercises beyond the intermediate level.

Timed Up & Go

This test is one of the most common balance tests used to assess general functional balance. You will need a standard chair for this test.

You will start from a seated position. Stand, walk three meters, turn around, walk back, and return to a seated position.

Performing this test in under 13.5 seconds indicates a pass. If you cannot perform this test in this amount of time, it suggests a higher risk of falling. It also shows that you should start with basic seated exercises before moving on to the more challenging exercises.

Practical Tips and Reminders

Safety is crucial when performing balance tests. If you're concerned about safely conducting these tests, consider seeing a physical therapist who can administer them in a clinical setting. If you're uncertain about your next steps after taking the balance tests, consulting a medical professional for guidance is advisable. It's important to ask questions rather than risk injury.

Regular testing and retesting are essential, as your condition can change over time. You might improve or experience setbacks, so adjusting your exercise plan is important. Regularly assessing your balance is a crucial part of this process. Balance tests are valuable for evaluating different aspects of balance and understanding your fall risk. This knowledge enables you to develop a personalized exercise plan suited to your strengths and abilities.

Having learned about common balance tests and how to perform them, let's move on to preparing for your exercises.

BEFORE YOU START

Even with balance exercises, it's crucial to warm-up and cool down, especially for seniors. Warming up prepares your muscles and joints, reducing the risk of injury and enhancing performance during exercise. Cooling down helps with recovery.

A BMC medical study showed that neuromuscular warm-ups and cool-downs significantly reduce injury risk, not just in seniors but also in young athletes and military recruits. Neuromuscular warm-ups involve stretches and movements that loosen muscles and ready the body for exercise. Skipping this step is tempting, but warming up is critical for a successful and safe exercise routine.

Consistency is vital not only in your exercise routine but also in your preparations. It's not enough to warm-up and cool down occasionally; these practices should be part of every session. Just as regular exercises build strength and improve balance over time, consistent warm-up and cool-down routines help prevent injuries and enhance the overall effectiveness of your workouts. Remember to be patient with yourself as you establish these habits. Getting used to new routines takes time, but your body will gradually adapt.

Maximizing Training Benefits

Developing a consistent balance routine, which includes warming up and cooling down, is crucial. Remember, improving balance and flexibility is a gradual process that requires time and persistent effort.

Don't be discouraged if progress seems slow. It's more about regularity than the duration of each session. Our goal is to retrain muscles and build strength in critical areas. You'll achieve better results with short, regular exercise multiple times a week rather than a single, long session followed by days of rest. Ten minutes a day, five days a week, with two rest days, is an excellent start.

As you get comfortable with ten-minute sessions, gradually increase the duration until you reach 20-30 minutes daily. This consistent, incremental approach is ideal for seeing improvements over time.

Managing Expectations

It's essential to recognize that balance exercises aren't a cure-all. They can significantly aid in maintaining independence and an active lifestyle for many people, but setting realistic goals is key to tracking progress. If your goals are too ambitious or unrealistic, it's easy to become discouraged. Remember, seeing the results of any physical activity takes time, but with consistent effort, progress will happen. Consistency and patience are vital in this journey.

Setting and achieving smaller, attainable goals is an effective way to monitor your progress, see how much you've improved, and maintain motivation. Completing these smaller milestones can boost your confidence and motivation, encouraging you to stick with your exercise routine.

Exercise Recommendations and Approvals

It's not always true that more exercise is better, especially for seniors with unique needs, limitations, and capabilities. The CDC provides guidelines for the type and amount of exercise suitable for seniors. Any physical activity is beneficial, as regular movement is necessary to maintain flexibility and fitness. For those over 65, the CDC recommends 150 minutes of moderate activity weekly. Combining 10 minutes of balance exercises with 20 minutes of walking or light exercise daily aligns well with these guidelines.

For those capable of high-intensity activities like running or hiking, only 75 minutes per week is needed. It's crucial to include both muscle-strengthening and balance exercises in your routine. To complement balance exercises, you can incorporate walking with your stretches for well-rounded training that includes cardiovascular exercise.

Adjusting Workouts

Avoid exercises that make you uncomfortable or cause pain. You can make modifications to reduce the difficulty or strain of a move. This guide will cover ways to adjust exercises for various limitations. Knowing your limits and not pushing beyond them is crucial. It's safer to err on the side of caution. If uncertain about an exercise, start with its modified, easier version and gradually increase the difficulty as you become more comfortable.

Seeking Professional Advice

If you have specific health concerns that might affect your exercise routine or are unsure about any aspect of this guide, consult a medical professional. Your doctor or physical therapist can provide advice to enhance your exercise success and minimize injury risk. It's generally wise for you to inform your doctor about new exercise plans, as they can offer helpful tips and ensure your routine is safe for your health needs.

Utilizing Video for Technique Assessment

Videos can be highly beneficial in various ways. Firstly, use the videos accompanying this book to check and improve your form. Correct form is essential to avoid injuries. If you're unsure about your technique, consult a professional. You can record yourself and compare your form with the videos to learn how to perform the exercises safely.

Additionally, videos can be a motivational tool by visually tracking your skill and ability improvement over time. Remember, improving your balance and strength is an ongoing process with continuous room for growth. Putting in this extra effort can significantly enhance the benefits you gain from your exercises.

How to Perform a Rep

You'll encounter a few key terms when starting your exercise journey: sets, repetitions (reps), and rest intervals. We will go through each term below.

A "**rep**" refers to one complete cycle of an exercise. For instance, in a squat, you start standing, lower into the squat position, and then stand back up–that's one rep. Therefore, performing the exercise move three times equals three reps.

A "**set**" refers to a group of reps done together. For example, ten squats might make one set. If you're instructed to do two sets of squats, you'll do 20 squats in total.

A "**rest interval**" is the break you take between sets. Depending on the exercise, these can be short or long. They're crucial for allowing your body to recover before the next set.

This guide explains how to complete one rep of each exercise successfully. Typically, you'll aim for 8-12 reps with 30-60 second rest intervals between each set. Focus on correct form over the number of reps and sets. If you can't do a complete set initially, that's okay; you can work up to it. Proper form is essential to prevent injury and achieve effective results. It's better to do fewer reps correctly than more reps incorrectly. In addition to proper form, good breathing is also incredibly important.

Breathing

When doing any form of strength training, it's crucial to breathe correctly for optimal performance and safety. Inhale through your nose before the muscle-lengthening (eccentric) phase and exhale through your mouth during the muscle-shortening (concentric) phase. For instance, in a squat, inhale as you lower and exhale as you rise. Similarly, during a pushup, inhale as you descend and exhale as you push up. Avoid holding your breath, as it can elevate blood pressure. Instead, focus on deep breathing, promoting relaxation and lowering blood pressure. With consistent practice, proper breathing during exercise becomes instinctive.

Warm-Up and Cool Down

Warming up and cooling down is crucial for a successful balance exercise routine. These steps ensure you get the most benefit from your exercises and don't take much time. Spending about five minutes on simple warm-up and cool-down activities can significantly reduce the risk of injury during workouts and improve the effectiveness of your exercises.

When engaging in warm-up and cool-down exercises, select activities appropriate for your fitness level. If there's a risk of instability during these exercises, it's important to have someone nearby to assist you, or choose an easier option.

Injury Mitigation

Warming up boosts oxygen flow to muscles and joints, preparing them for activity and making them less likely to tear or strain when put under stress. It also raises your body temperature and heart rate, making your body more ready for exercise. Cooling down gradually brings your body back to its resting state. Both practices enhance suppleness and potentially expand your range of motion, further protecting you from injuries and strains during physical activities.

Effective Warm-Up Techniques

Warming up prepares your body for more intense activities. It includes dynamic stretching and raising your body temperature. Gradually increasing your heart rate enhances blood flow and circulation, preparing your body for exercise. It also helps you mentally focus for the workout.

One of the first things you must do is get your heart rate and body temperature up. The easiest way to do this is through brisk walking. A few times up and down the stairs is highly effective as well.

Dynamic Stretching

A dynamic stretch is a move that will help you limber up your joints and muscles. Let's take a look at some of the most common and easy dynamic stretches:

- **Arms circles**: Stand or sit with your feet shoulder-width apart and extend your arms to the sides at shoulder height, palms facing down. Begin moving your arms in small, slow circles. Gradually increase the circle size for 20 rotations. If you require additional support for balance, do this exercise near a countertop or a stable surface.

- **Hip circles**: Start standing upright with your feet slightly wider than shoulder-width apart and your knees softly bent. Place your hands on your hips. Begin by slowly rotating your hips, making large, circular motions. Complete a set of rotations in one direction, then reverse the motion, rotating your hips in the opposite direction. Complete 10 reps in each direction.

- **Roll downs**: Stand with feet hip-width apart, spine straight, and shoulders relaxed. Inhale, engaging your abdominal muscles. Exhale and tuck your chin, letting your arms dangle and rolling your spine down vertebra by vertebra, knees slightly bent. Go as far as comfortable. With your tailbone tucked and abdominal muscles engaged, inhale deeply. Exhale and slowly roll back up, starting from your lower back, using your core to realign each vertebra, and finishing with your head.

Some other easy warm-up techniques include:

- **Seated roll downs:** In a seated position, perform a roll down, bending forward as far as comfortable. Exhale and roll back up.

- **Shoulder rolls:** In a seated or standing position, roll your shoulders forward in a circular motion, keeping your back straight and your core engaged. Do rolls forward and backward.

- **Shrugs:** In a seated or standing position, inhale and bring your shoulders up to your ears as high as possible. Exhale and lower back down.

- **Neck circles:** In a seated position, slowly rotate your head around in a circular motion. Ensure you complete circles in both directions.

- **Ankle rolls:** While seated, extend one leg forward so the foot is off the ground. Slowly rotate your foot in a circular motion around the ankle joint.

- **Seated twists:** Sitting upright with your back straight and your eyes forward, slowly rotate your torso as far as is comfortable in one direction before returning to the center and repeating in the other direction.

- **Marching on the spot:** Seated or standing, march on the spot by raising one knee and the opposing arm in a controlled manner.

- **Star steps (star jumps but without the jump):** Seated or standing, step one foot out to the side while simultaneously raising both arms above your head and touching fingers. Repeat with the other leg.

- **Brisk walking:** Go for a short walk at a pace slightly above normal walking pace with the goal of increasing your heart rate.

- **Stair climbing:** Ascending and descending a flight of stairs a few times, again, to raise your heart rate. Be conscious of your current balance and mobility.

- **Seated knee extension:** While seated, extend one leg out in front of you, hinging at the knee. Every part of your body above your knee should be unmoved.

- **Seated heel raises:** An excellent way to warm-up your calves, while seated with your back straight and eyes forward, lift your heels off the ground, keeping the balls of your feet firmly planted on the floor.

- **Standing leg curls:** Holding onto something for support, stand with feet hip-width apart, eyes forward and back straight. Raise one foot behind you, pivoting at the knee and keeping your thigh unmoved. Raise as high as is comfortable.

- **Standing supported hip side raise:** Holding something for support, raise one leg out to the side while keeping your back straight. Return your leg to standing in a controlled manner.

- **Standing small hip swing forward-backward:** Similar to the side raise, although holding a chair for support to the side. Swing one leg at a time forward and backward in a controlled manner.

Guiding a Safe Cool Down

Cooling down is a low-impact process that is the counterpart to warming up. It includes gentle movements and static stretches, often lighter versions of your warm-up exercises, as well as certain breathing techniques, to reduce your body temperature and heart rate gradually. The aim is to smoothly transition your body from active to resting, helping prevent sudden strain after your body cools down too quickly. While cooling down is a simpler process than warming up, it is equally important in ensuring a safe and effective transition from physical activity, aiding in the recovery and relaxation of your muscles.

Some simple cool down exercises include:

- **Hamstring stretch:** Can be performed seated or standing; place one heel on the ground in front of you, extending the leg while the other bends slightly at the knee. Keeping your back straight, bend at the hip to bring your chest slightly toward your thigh.

- **Seated glute stretch:** While sitting on a chair, raise your left leg and cross your left ankle on top of your right knee. Keeping your back straight, bend forward slightly until you feel a stretch in your left glute. Repeat with the other leg.

- **Standing hip flexor stretch:** Step forward from a standing position, bending your front knee slightly while keeping your back leg straight. Push your hips forward to feel a stretch in your hip. Maintain an upright chest, hold the stretch for a few seconds, and return to the starting position by pushing through your front foot.

- **Pectoral stretch:** Stand in an open doorway with your arms raised to the side, bent 90 degrees at the elbow with your palms facing forward. Step one foot forward and gently press against the door frame with your arms to feel a stretch across your pectorals.

- **Overhead tricep stretch:** Raise your shoulders toward your ears, then draw them down and back, extending your right arm to the ceiling and bending at the elbow to rest your right palm near the center of your back with your middle finger along your spine. Place your left hand on your right elbow to help feel the stretch.

- **Shoulder stretch:** Bring your right arm across your body with a slightly bent elbow, using your left hand to guide the movement as you press your arm into your chest and toward the left.

- **Pursed-lip breathing:** This effectively slows down your breathing rate while increasing the effectiveness of each breath. Lower your shoulders, close your eyes, and inhale through your nose for 2 seconds before slowly exhaling through your pursed lips for 4-6 seconds without forcing the air out. Repeat this until your breathing has slowed.

Essential Exercise Equipment

This exercise guide is designed to be accessible, requiring only a few basic items. A chair is a key piece of equipment for both sitting and standing exercises. An exercise mat is recommended for comfort during floor exercises, and these are found in most sporting goods stores. A tennis ball can also be handy for certain activities.

If you want to add more challenge to your workouts, consider incorporating an exercise ball for seated exercises. This is a large, inflatable ball that can enhance various routines. Additionally, using a light dumbbell for certain exercises, which will be specified later in the guide, can also increase the intensity of your workout. These items are optional and should be used only if you feel comfortable and have a safe space with support available. Now that we've laid the groundwork, let's get into the exercises.

SEATED EXERCISES

Seated exercises are a fantastic starting point for our guide because they are highly accessible and strongly emphasize safety. These exercises are ideal for beginners or those who need to start with lower intensity or modified movements. They are not only effective in improving balance but also in reducing the risk of falls.

What makes seated balance exercises particularly beneficial is their versatility. You can easily incorporate them into different parts of your day, allowing for more activity than you might usually undertake. While having a structured exercise routine is important, these exercises are adaptable enough to be performed at various times throughout the day.

These seated exercises are crucial in enhancing your balance, flexibility, and strength, vital to staying active and reducing fall risks in later years. Starting, even with modified versions, is an important stride toward autonomy and control over your well-being. We've carefully selected safe and adjustable exercises to suit a range of abilities.

All of our seated exercises, except for leaning down on elbow, can be modified by using an exercise ball instead of a chair. However, this modification increases the difficulty and risk, particularly if your balance is not yet well-developed. We recommend mastering all the exercises in this guide using a standard chair before trying them with an exercise ball. When you feel ready to attempt these exercises on an exercise ball, ensure you have someone nearby to assist you for safety.

In this guide, each exercise will be detailed with its difficulty level, instructions on how to perform it, and modifications.

Shifting Weight Side-to-Side

The side-to-side weight shift exercise is designed to improve balance and coordination by testing your proprioceptive and vestibular systems due to the weight shift from one side to the other. It's a simple yet effective exercise suitable for beginners.

To perform this exercise, sit upright in a chair with your back straight. Engage your core muscles, then slowly lean to one side, pausing for a few seconds, before returning to the center. Repeat the same movement on the other side. One rep involves leaning over to each side.

For those who find it challenging, the exercise can be modified by initially leaning only slightly to each side. As you build strength and balance, you can increase the extent of your lean. You can add more reps or sets to your routine to keep the exercise challenging as you progress.

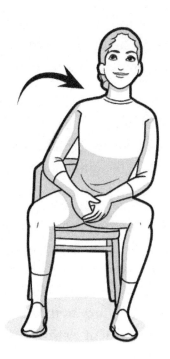
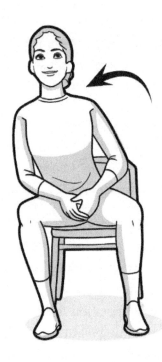

Shifting Weight Forward-to-Back

This exercise, similar to shifting weight side-to-side, is an effective way to enhance balance through the inner ear and sensory systems. It focuses on gently stretching and lengthening muscles to improve flexibility and range of motion.

This exercise is beneficial for transitioning safely between positions, minimizing the risk of imbalance. Ideal for beginners, this exercise can be tailored for comfort, including the option of using a cushion or pillow for back support.

To perform it, sit upright in a chair with your back straight. Engage your core muscles and lift your chest as you carefully shift your weight forward. Ensure your back remains straight and your breathing steady throughout the movement. Hold the forward position for a few seconds, then slowly return to the center, maintaining your posture. Perform this movement with control, especially when starting, to maximize its benefits.

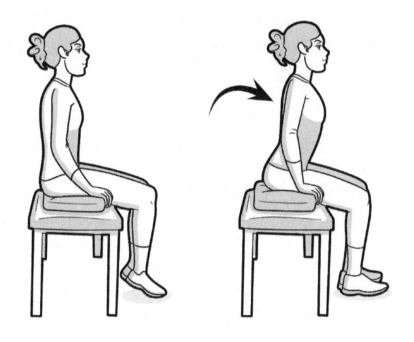

Trunk Circles

Trunk circles help engage and strengthen core muscles, including the abdominals. A stronger core can improve weight-bearing efficiency and enhance stability while standing. Additionally, performing trunk circles can increase the flexibility of the back muscles, making rotational movements and general mobility easier.

Rated as beginner, trunk circles can be modified to suit your comfort level. To make the exercise easier and reduce strain on the upper body, you can decrease the size of the circles.

To perform trunk circles, sit on a chair with your back straight. Throughout the exercise, focus on keeping your abdominal muscles tight, which helps engage the core properly. While seated, move your upper body in a circular motion. Begin with small circles and gradually increase their size as you become more comfortable with the movement. One rep consists of a circle in the clockwise and counterclockwise directions.

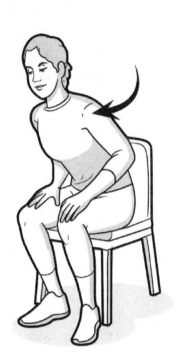
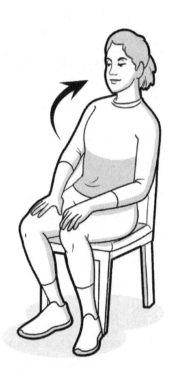

Lateral Trunk Flexion

Lateral trunk flexion is beneficial for strengthening the core muscles and lengthening the oblique and intercostal muscles. Strengthening these muscles enhances stability by improving weight distribution, which can help prevent falls. This movement is distinct from shifting weight side-to-side as you are flexing between the hip and ribcage.

This exercise is of beginner difficulty. To modify, you can adjust the depth of the movement according to your comfort and ability.

Lateral trunk flexion is excellent for improving both balance and posture, aiding in maintaining a proper seated position. To do this exercise, sit in a chair with your back straight and your core engaged. Then, gently tilt one shoulder toward the hip on the same side, creating a side-bending motion in your trunk.

If you find this movement challenging, you can enhance your stability by reaching your hand down the side of the chair. Aim to hold this position for about 5 seconds. Then, with controlled movements, return to the center before repeating the exercise on the other side for one rep.

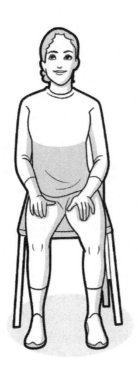
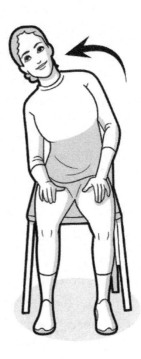

Leaning Down on Elbow

This exercise aims to strengthen the back, shoulder, and core muscles. This exercise is intermediate as it requires a certain degree of stability from the outset, so it's important to ensure you're strong and capable enough to perform it safely.

For those who find the exercise challenging, performing it on a softer surface like a bed or couch is beneficial. If additional support is needed, using a pillow to raise the elbow can provide extra support.

To do this move, sit upright on a couch or bed, engaging your core muscles. Then, lean sideways until you are resting on your elbow. Maintain this position for about 5 seconds before returning to an upright seated position. Repeat the movement on the other side for a complete rep. This exercise not only strengthens key muscle groups but also enhances your ability to control and stabilize your body, making it a valuable addition to your exercise routine.

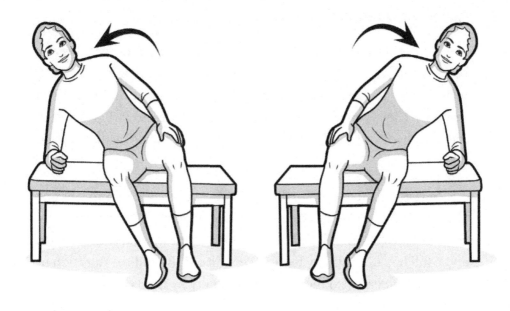

Leg Lift

This exercise primarily targets the hip flexors and secondarily the quadriceps. It engages the abdominal muscles, contributing to overall leg and core strength.

To perform a leg lift, sit with your back straight, feet directly below your knees, and use your hands for support. Lift your leg 6 to 10 inches off the ground, aiming to hold the position for about 5 seconds. Then, gently lower your leg back to the ground and repeat the movement with the other leg. A lift with each leg constituting one rep.

Suitable for beginners, the exercise can be modified to fit your abilities. If the entire movement is too challenging, lift your leg only a couple of inches or hold the lift for a shorter time. As you gain strength and confidence, gradually increase the lift height and the duration of the hold. You can also increase the difficulty by not holding onto the chair with your hands.

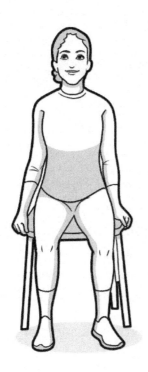
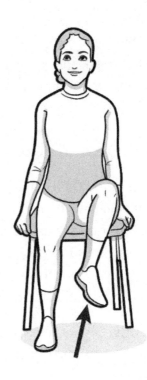

Hip Abduction Side Kicks

This movement primarily targets the hip abductor muscles in the outer thigh and gluteal region. These muscles are crucial for movements involving the leg's separation from the body's midline. The exercise can improve hip stability by strengthening these muscles, which are essential for weight-bearing activities and maintaining balance during daily movements.

To perform this exercise, start in a seated position with your legs about shoulder-width apart. Lift one foot off the ground, slowly kick your leg outward to the side, and then bring it back to your body. This move not only works your hip muscles but also allows you to feel a stretch during the movement. This beginner-level exercise can be modified by adjusting the range of motion at which you perform it.

For the best results, keep your torso straight and motionless to ensure the focus remains on your hip muscles. Complete once on both legs for one rep.

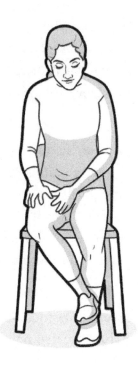
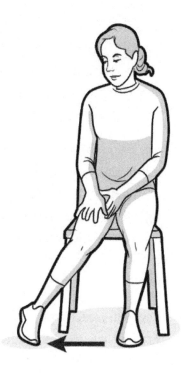

Reach With Clasped Hands

This exercise is designed to enhance coordination while working the core and shoulders. It offers flexibility in terms of difficulty adjustment. To make it easier, you can reduce the distance you reach. Try reaching out to the sides instead of just forward for a more challenging variation.

To perform this move, sit on a chair and clasp your hands together in your lap. Ensure your back is straight and your core muscles are engaged. Then, extend your clasped hands straight in front of you, reaching only as far as possible while maintaining stability. It's crucial to avoid overreaching to prevent the risk of falling. Keep your hands clasped throughout the exercise to ensure steady and controlled movement.

Once you reach out, hold the position for 5 seconds. Then, with care, return to your starting position. This exercise not only strengthens your upper body but also helps in maintaining upper body stability and control.

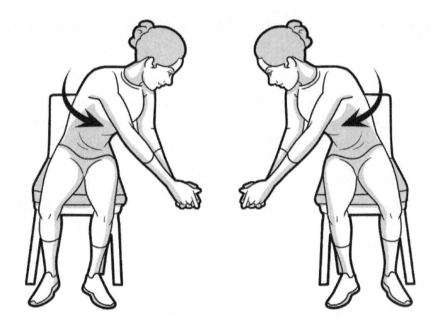

Reaching *This move necessitates a partner!*

This is an exercise that enhances flexibility and stability. It's slightly more challenging than reaching with clasped hands, requiring coordination both individually and with your partner.

Sit on a chair or another flat surface. Have your partner stand in front of you, holding a ball at various distances and heights. Reach for the ball as far as you comfortably can without compromising your stability. After reaching out, return to your initial sitting position.

To make this exercise more manageable, your partner can adjust the speed and distance at which they move the ball. If you're new to this exercise, start with slower movements at closer distances. As your confidence and ability improve, your partner can gradually increase the speed and extend the distance of the ball's positioning.

This exercise helps improve physical abilities and enhances coordination, making it a valuable and interactive component of your exercise routine.

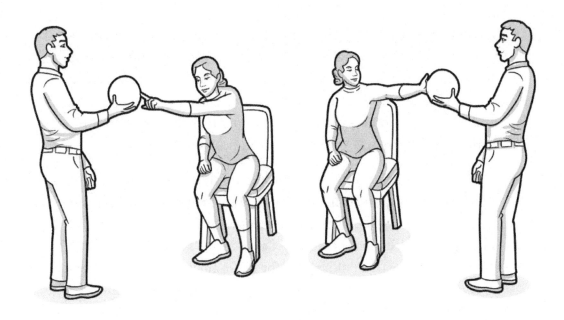

STANDING EXERCISES

Standing exercises are highly beneficial, particularly for seniors, as they enhance balance and reduce the risk of falls. Research suggests that standing for at least 45 minutes daily can lower mortality risk among seniors. While some of these movements are simple and straightforward, others present more of a challenge, effectively working various muscle groups to actively promote better health.

Unlike sitting exercises, standing routines activate different muscle groups, especially in the lower body, which is crucial for better balance and stability. This can significantly lower the risk of falls and injuries. Our selection of standing exercises caters to various skill and strength levels, with modifications for different abilities. This variety allows for a personalized approach to exercise, catering to individual needs and interests.

Prioritizing safety, the exercises we recommend are particularly beneficial for seniors, as they not only improve balance and strength but also facilitate daily activities like chores. An active lifestyle fostered through these exercises is essential for maintaining independence in later years.

Our guide aims to ensure the safe execution of these exercises and to illustrate their impact on daily life. While these exercises may initially present challenges, persistence is key. As they become more manageable over time, noticeable improvements in daily activities will occur.

Weight Shifting Front-to-Back

Front-to-back weight shifting improves standing balance, enhances proprioception, and promotes stable and correct posture. It's a beginner-friendly exercise and can be modified to suit individual needs.

For those new to this exercise, using a chair for support can be helpful. Place it in front of you to hold onto if you feel unsteady. As you gain confidence and stability, you can gradually reduce your reliance on the chair. The ultimate goal is to perform this balance exercise without needing any support.

To do the exercise, stand with your feet shoulder-width apart. Begin by shifting your weight forward, allowing your heels to lift slightly off the ground. Then, shift your weight backward, letting your toes lift slightly. This forward and backward movement helps train your body to maintain balance during shifts in weight distribution, which is crucial for stability in daily activities.

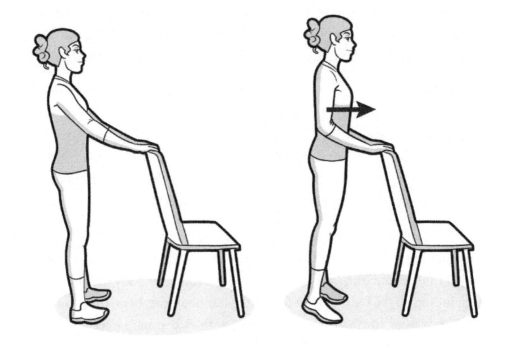

Heel Raises

Heel raises are an effective exercise for enhancing stability while standing and walking. They primarily focus on strengthening the calf muscles, which play a significant role in stabilizing the ankle joint.

This exercise is suitable for beginners and can be modified as needed. If you're new to heel raises or need extra support, it's advisable to start with a chair in front of you for balance. As you become more comfortable and stable, you can perform the exercise without the chair. For those who can easily do this move, holding a light hand weight can add intensity to the exercise.

To do heel raises, stand with your back straight and feet hip-width apart. Keep your hands at your sides, but if you feel unstable, feel free to hold onto the chair for support. Lift your body up so you're standing on the balls of your feet with your heels raised off the ground. Then, slowly lower back to standing, with that cycle being one rep. This exercise not only strengthens your lower legs but also helps in maintaining balance during various activities.

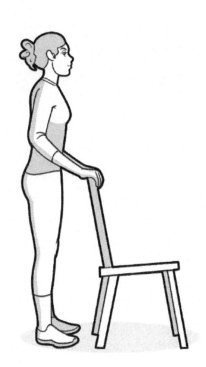
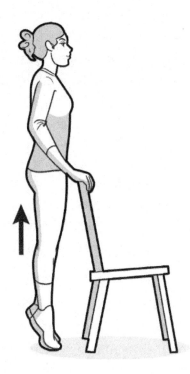

Hip Abduction

The hip abduction exercise primarily targets the muscles on the outer thigh and the gluteal region, particularly the gluteus medius and minimus. These muscles are crucial for moving the leg away from the body's midline. By strengthening these muscles, hip abduction exercises can improve balance, as these muscles are vital for stabilizing the pelvis during activities like walking and standing on one leg.

Classified as an intermediate-level exercise, hip abduction requires a degree of balance. If needed, you can begin by using a chair for support and gradually move away from relying on it as your balance improves, but only do so when you feel it's safe.

To perform this exercise, stand with your feet together, keeping a chair nearby for necessary support. Shift your weight onto one leg and simultaneously lift the other leg out to the side. You should focus on maintaining proper posture while extending your leg rather than lifting it as high as possible. Keep your leg in line with your body. After extending, bring it back to the center and repeat the movement with the other leg for one rep.

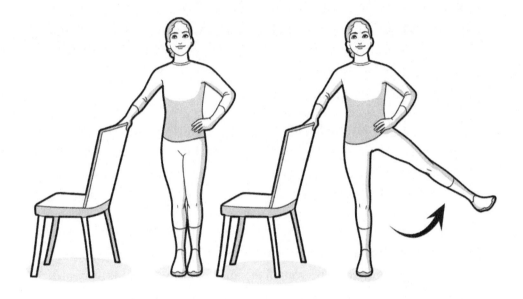

Kickback Hip Extension

Kickback hip extensions are primarily aimed at strengthening the gluteal muscles and hamstrings. This exercise involves extending the leg backward and activating the buttocks and rear thigh muscles. The exercise contributes to lower body strength, which is important for overall stability. It may offer some benefits in hip joint flexibility, although this is not its primary purpose.

Classified as an intermediate exercise, starting with a chair for balance is advisable, especially if you're uncertain about your stability. To make the exercise easier, you can slow the movement and reduce how much you extend your leg.

To do the movement, face a chair and stand straight with your feet together. Gradually lift one leg behind you, keeping your posture straight, hips aligned with your feet, and avoiding leaning forward. Then, return to your starting position. Repeat this movement with the other leg for one complete rep. Keeping your hips aligned with your feet throughout is crucial, even if it means you can only go back a couple of inches.

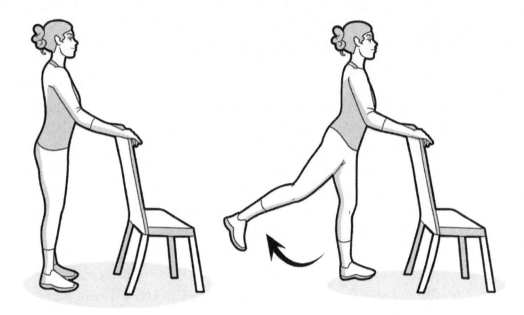

Step-Up

The step-up exercise is a functional movement designed to enhance overall stability, particularly during activities like climbing stairs or navigating uneven surfaces. It targets core and lower body muscles, including the quadriceps, hamstrings, and glutes, which are crucial for maintaining balance.

This exercise is classified as intermediate, depending on your ability, as it demands both strength and coordination. To make it safer, complete the movement near something sturdy you can hold onto for support. Doing this on the first step of a staircase while holding onto the handrail works perfectly.

To perform the movement, find a stable step or platform. Stand with your feet hip-width apart and step one foot onto the step. Shift your weight forward onto your leading leg and push, rising onto the step with support from the trailing leg. Stand up straight with both feet on the step. Then, step back down, leading with the same leg and maintaining control throughout the movement. Complete the step-up with both legs for one rep. This exercise simulates real-life movements, improving your functional fitness.

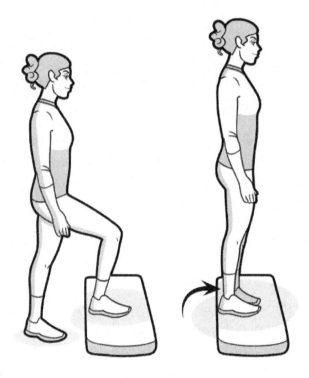

Sit to Stand

This exercise primarily aims to strengthen the lower body, particularly the quadriceps, glutes, and hamstrings. Strengthening these muscles can enhance a safer transition from sitting to standing and can, therefore, reduce balance-related falls and injuries.

This exercise involves moving from seated to standing, making it an intermediate-level activity. You can start by using sturdy support for assistance and then gradually progress to performing the exercise without support when you feel ready.

Begin by sitting in a chair with your feet planted flat on the floor, shoulder-width apart. Sit in the middle of the chair with your back straight. Shift your weight forward, slowly transferring your weight from your buttocks to your feet as you rise off the chair. Stand up straight at the top with your core and glutes engaged before sitting back down in a controlled motion to complete the rep. This exercise is beneficial for improving functional movements used in daily activities.

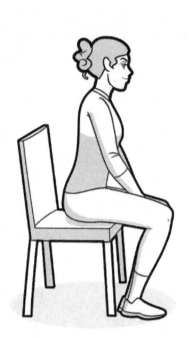
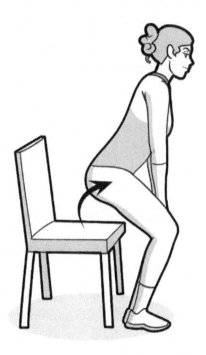

One-Leg Stand

This movement primarily focuses on enhancing balance and strengthening the legs, as well as the joints in the lower body. Improved leg strength and balance can ease the transition from sitting to standing and facilitate the safer execution of more complex, coordinated activities.

Additionally, performing the one-leg stand contributes to better posture. Maintaining balance on one leg requires proper body alignment, which helps train the postural muscles. This can lead to more secure and effortless movements in daily activities, especially those requiring coordination and balance.

This exercise is somewhat challenging as it requires a good level of balance. If you find it difficult, you can use a chair for additional support or shorten the duration of each stance. To perform the exercise, stand with your feet together, facing a wall. Extend your arms so that your fingertips lightly touch the wall for balance. Keep your hips level as you raise one leg in front of you to 90 degrees, holding for up to 15 seconds, then slowly return to the starting position and repeat with the other leg.

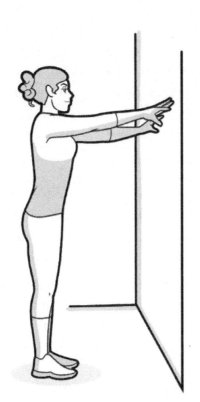 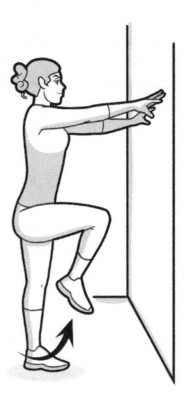

Lunge

The lunge is a beneficial leg exercise targeting key muscle groups like the glutes, hamstrings, quads, and calves. It is known for improving balance, strength, and stability. This exercise requires a strong core engagement due to its inherent instability, and it also enhances hip flexibility and mobility, which is essential for daily activities. The added instability makes the lunge a challenging exercise.

To do a lunge, start by standing straight with your feet hip-width apart, looking forward, and your arms either on your hips or holding something stable for support. Step forward with one foot, bending both knees to form 90-degree angles, ensuring the front knee doesn't go past the toes, and keeping the back knee a couple of inches off the ground. Keep your weight mainly on the front leg while the back leg supports. Maintain an upright chest and forward gaze, then push through your front foot to return to the starting position.

Alternate the lunge with the other leg for one complete repetition. Hold a light dumbbell with each hand by your side for an added challenge.

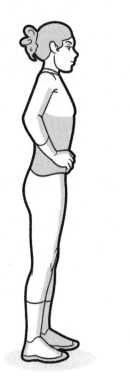

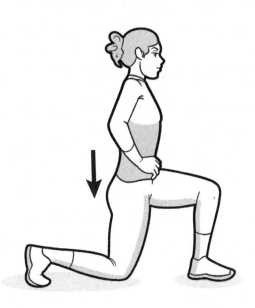

Lateral Lunge

This exercise engages muscles that are often underutilized, significantly enhancing overall strength and stability. It primarily targets the inner and outer thighs (adductors and abductors), hips, glutes, quads, hamstrings, and calves. Additionally, it works the core, as stability is crucial while performing the exercise, making it a challenging yet effective workout.

To perform this exercise, begin by standing up straight with your feet hip-width apart, toes forward, eyes and head facing forward, and arms relaxed at your sides. Activate your core and take a step to the right with your right foot, transferring your weight onto it. Lower into a squat by bending your right knee and pushing your hips back while keeping your left leg straight and both feet pointing forward; extending your arms in front may help with balance.

Maintain an open chest and neutral spine, then push through your right foot to stand up and repeat the movement with your left leg for a full rep.

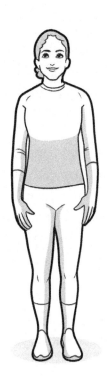

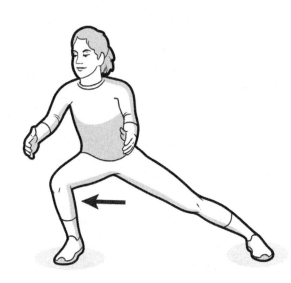

Standing Knee Lift

This exercise mainly targets the quadriceps and glutes, but it's especially effective for strengthening the stabilizing muscles around the knee and ankle. It is a challenging exercise with a higher risk of falling, so make sure to do it near something stable for support.

To do this exercise, start by standing upright with your feet hip-width apart, shoulders pulled back, core engaged, and arms at your sides. Gradually lift one foot off the ground, bending your knee until it reaches chest level, then hold your knee with your hands and gently pull it closer to your chest. Be mindful of your physical limits and avoid pushing yourself too hard.

Maintaining balance is easier if you focus on a stationary object ahead. If you start to lose balance, gently lower your foot to the ground and try again. Initially, lift your knee to a 90-degree angle, and as you grow more confident, gradually bring it closer to your chest. Aim to hold this position for 20-30 seconds on each leg.

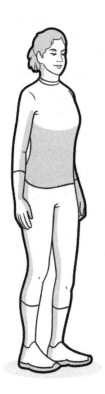
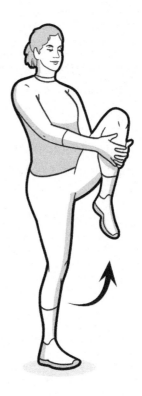

Squat

This movement is a comprehensive balance exercise that targets the core, lower body, and back muscles, enhancing overall stability and balance. It's particularly beneficial for improving the transition from sitting to standing and can aid in performing daily tasks like safely lifting and carrying items.

The squat involves strength and coordination, so it's considered a challenging exercise. Keep a chair or other sturdy surface within reach to ensure safety, especially when starting out or if stability is a concern. Beginners can modify the squat by not going as low.

To perform the squat, stand with your feet hip-width apart, distributing your weight evenly between the balls and heels of your feet, toes pointing forward. Push your hips back, bending at the knees and ankles, and press your knees slightly outward. Lower into a squat, keeping heels and toes grounded, chest up, and shoulders back. Go no lower than 90 degrees. Hold the squat for 2 seconds, then reverse the movement to return to standing. Remember to engage your core and glutes before beginning.

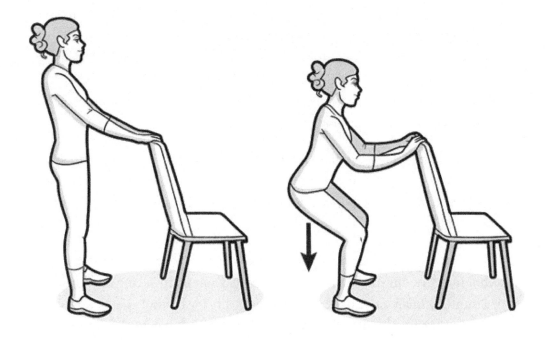

Bicep Curls for Balance

Bicep curls while balancing is an effective exercise for enhancing coordination and balance. It engages your upper body through the bicep curl while challenging your lower body and core stability as you balance on one leg. This dual-action exercise can improve steadiness during everyday activities, especially those requiring simultaneous upper and lower body coordination.

This exercise is challenging due to the coordination and balance involved. If you're new, begin without weight and use a chair for support. As you progress, you can gradually introduce a light dumbbell.

To execute the movement, stand with your feet together, holding the dumbbell in one hand with your palm facing forward. Simultaneously raise the heel of the opposite leg behind you, bending at the knee to create a 90-degree angle. Hold this position for 2 seconds before gently lowering your leg and arm back to the starting position. Switch to the other arm and leg to complete one rep.

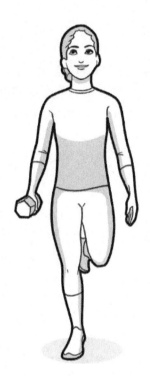
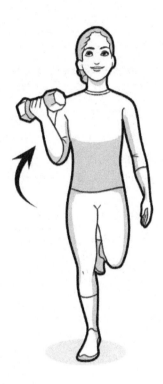

WALKING EXERCISES

Staying active is crucial for health, particularly in older age. Engaging in high-intensity activities is not necessary; rather, the focus should be on moderate, achievable exercises that support and maintain our independence. The CDC underscores the importance of activity for seniors, advising those 65 and older to aim for at least 150 minutes of moderate exercise weekly, such as walking.

There's also a growing recognition among seniors of the importance of exercise for both physical and mental health. A survey by AARP shows that most seniors understand the health benefits of walking.

Walking exercises are particularly beneficial. They're simple, adaptable, and can significantly improve physical and mental health. Gradual progression and realistic goal-setting can keep you motivated, enhancing your balance and strength, which are vital for sustaining independence and minimizing fall risks. Beyond physical health, walking promotes mental clarity and emotional well-being, with regular walkers often experiencing heightened happiness and reduced depression symptoms.

Tailored specifically for seniors, the walking exercises in this guide offer safety and efficacy, with modifications available for varying levels of ability. Always prioritize safety and consult a physical therapist if you have any concerns about the exercises.

For these exercises, a single rep includes a step with each leg. If you are doing an exercise like sideways walking, it makes sense to complete all the steps of a set in one direction before completing the remainder in the other direction to save you from staying in the same spot. Given that 8-12 reps of some of these exercises might not be much, a good goal is to aim for 30-60 seconds of activity per set for each exercise.

Sideways Walk

Sideways walking is a practical and beneficial exercise for seniors, targeting the muscles used in daily activities to strengthen and improve flexibility. Enhanced muscle function from this exercise contributes significantly to better balance.

As a beginner-level exercise, sideways walking is accessible for most seniors and doesn't require much strength. Nonetheless, safety is essential. If you're uncertain about your balance, stay close to a wall for support. Starting near a wall is wise to catch yourself if you feel unsteady at any point.

To do this exercise, stand up straight with your feet together. Move laterally by stepping to the side with one foot, followed by the other, moving with control. Ensure to walk in both directions to maintain balance in muscle development.

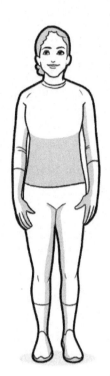
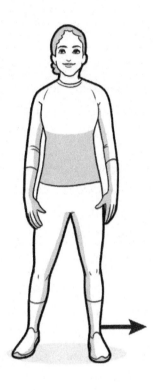

Heel-to-Toe Walk

The heel-to-toe walk is an effective exercise for improving dynamic balance. This is particularly important as many falls occur while in motion, and exercises that test regular movement patterns and your proprioceptive system can help prevent these falls.

This exercise is beginner-friendly and can be adapted to fit most seniors. If balance is a concern, you can use a walking aid or perform the exercise alongside a wall for additional support. With practice, as your balance improves, you may need less support and can move away from the wall.

To begin the heel-to-toe walk, stand up straight with your feet together. Step forward, placing your right heel directly in front of the toes of your left foot. Continue by placing your left heel in front of the toes of your right foot. Keep your gaze and head straight ahead to help maintain balance.

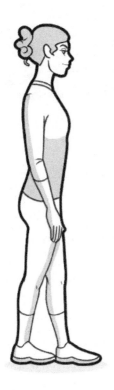
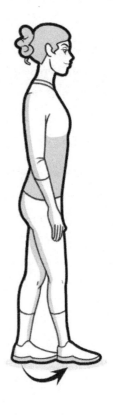

Heel Walk

Heel walking is an excellent exercise for seniors to improve balance and strengthen lower leg muscles, particularly the tibialis anterior (shin muscle.) This exercise enhances stability and proprioception, reducing the risk of falls, and can be particularly beneficial in promoting a steadier gait.

Before attempting heel walking, considered an intermediate activity, ensure you're comfortable performing the more basic exercises. As an intermediate exercise, you can modify the movement by staying close to a supportive surface like a wall or chair. Initially, you may also choose to heel walk with one foot at a time and the other foot flat on the floor.

To begin heel walking, stand with your back straight and feet slightly apart. Lift the toes of both feet so only your heels are on the ground, and proceed to walk forward on your heels for a few steps. After a few heel-only steps, turn carefully and return to your starting point.

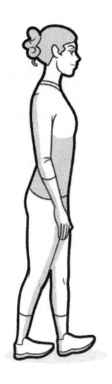
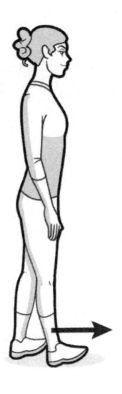

Toe Walk

Toe walking effectively targets the muscles in the feet and calves, which are crucial for balance but often overlooked in daily activities. It helps build muscle strength in these areas and contributes to static and dynamic balance. While primarily focusing on the lower legs, toe walking also engages core muscles, enhancing trunk stability.

Classified as an intermediate exercise, toe walking can challenge your balance and should be approached with caution. For added safety, stay close to a wall or chair to provide support, and walk a shorter distance to begin.

To initiate toe walking, stand with your feet together, engaging your core and glutes. Lift yourself onto your tiptoes, using a chair or wall for balance if necessary. While remaining on your toes, carefully walk a few steps forward, then turn and walk back to your starting point.

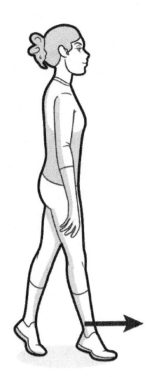
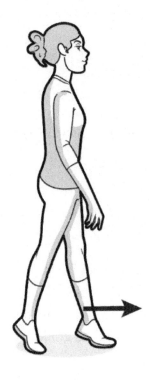

Backward Walk

Backward walking is a multifaceted exercise that works the hamstrings, quadriceps, and calves. Beyond physical benefits, it enhances cognitive functions like spatial awareness and coordination.

It is considered a beginner to intermediate exercise. Still, having someone accompany you for safety when performing this move is advisable. Additionally, performing the exercise near a wall or with a chair nearby is recommended for added support.

To perform backward walking, begin by standing with your feet together. Carefully take a few steps back, pause, turn around, and walk backward to your starting position. As your confidence and balance improve, you can gradually increase the distance of your walk.

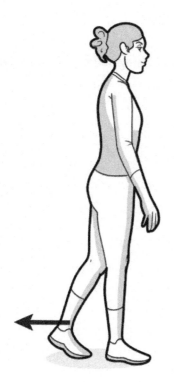
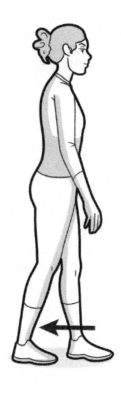

Balance Walk

Balance walking is an effective exercise designed to enhance your ability to control weight distribution on one leg, thus improving balance. This skill is handy for performing more complex movements safely and efficiently.

Classified as intermediate in difficulty, balance walking can be modified for beginners. Hold onto something for support and lift your legs only slightly to make it less challenging.

To execute balance walking, stand upright with your feet hip-width apart and extend your arms to the sides at shoulder height. Keep your head up and your gaze forward rather than looking down. Walk forward and pause briefly each time you lift a leg, holding the raised knee position for a moment before stepping forward. Focus on smooth, controlled movements. The goal is to raise the knee so your leg is at 90 degrees but manage your ability accordingly.

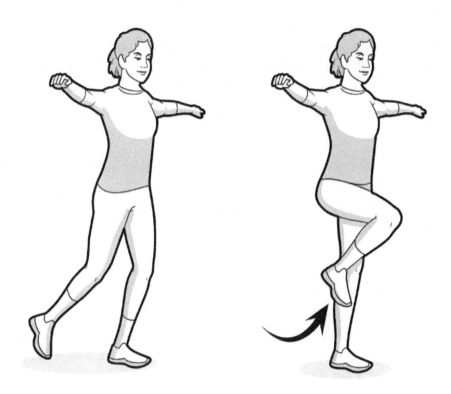

Head Turning Walk

Head turning while walking improves postural balance by training the body to maintain upright stability and proper weight distribution, even when the head is turned in various directions. It is particularly effective in enhancing dynamic balance and improving the vestibular system.

Classified as intermediate to difficult, this exercise requires walking coordination while simultaneously moving your head. Due to the complexity and increased risk of disorientation, it's recommended to have someone present for safety and ensure the area is clear of obstacles.

Begin by standing straight with your feet slightly apart. Walk forward normally. As you walk, turn your head alternately to the left and then to the right with every other step. After completing the side-to-side head turns, look upwards and downwards with every other step as you continue walking.

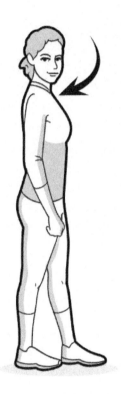
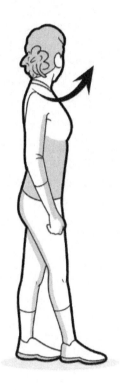

Serpentine Walk

The serpentine walk, also known as the figure 8 walk, is a dynamic exercise that improves balance by requiring constant weight shifting and adjustments. While it works your lower body, as with any walking exercise, the main benefit is the coordination needed to complete it.

This exercise is rated intermediate. To make it more manageable when starting, move slowly with gentle turns. This move should be performed in open spaces, allowing for the natural flow of the serpentine pattern.

To do the walk, take a few steps in one direction, then smoothly transition to the opposite direction, creating a flowing, snake-like path as you proceed. Focus on controlled, fluid movements to trace the imaginary figure 8 on the ground.

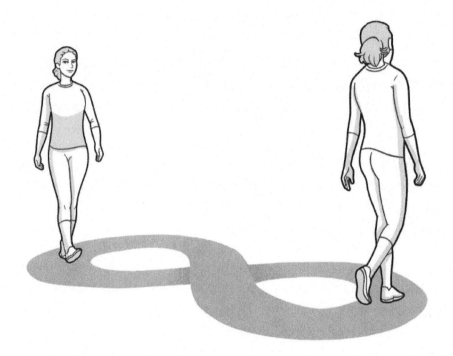

Grapevine Walk

Grapevine walking is an advanced exercise that targets overall stability and the ability to coordinate complex body movements without losing balance. It's particularly beneficial for enhancing the agility required during standing, sitting, and walking transitions.

Given its complexity, grapevine walking is considered challenging. Having a companion nearby when you're first learning this exercise and performing it in a clutter-free area is advisable. To simplify the movement, slow down.

To begin grapevine walking, stand with your feet shoulder-width apart. Keeping your hips in line, step your left foot across your body so your legs are crossed. Next, step your right foot to the right so your feet are uncrossed and shoulder-width apart again. Then, repeat the process, stepping your left foot behind your body instead of in front. This move requires coordination, but with some practice, it is a great exercise to improve your balance.

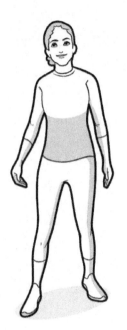
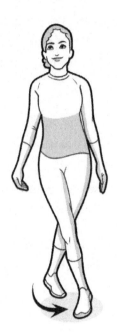
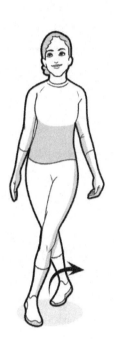

Ball Toss Walk

Ball toss walking is an engaging exercise that enhances balance and stability while honing hand-eye coordination. It teaches you to synchronize movements of your hands and feet, which is crucial for maintaining dynamic balance—keeping upright while your attention is divided between different tasks.

This exercise is challenging and suitable for those looking to advance their coordination. It can be done solo or with a partner. Pause after each step to catch the ball to make it less difficult. The goal is to walk seamlessly while throwing and catching the ball. The perfect ball for this exercise is a tennis ball or a small inflatable exercise ball.

The exercise can be varied in two other ways: 1) if solo, walk while bouncing the ball on the ground to focus on coordination between hand movements and steps, and 2) if working with a partner, pass the ball sideways to them while you both walk at a controlled pace.

Regardless of the method, the goal is maintaining balance while focusing on the ball, improving your multitasking ability.

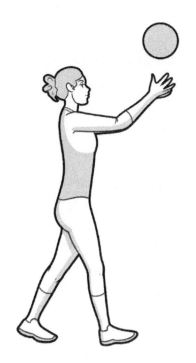
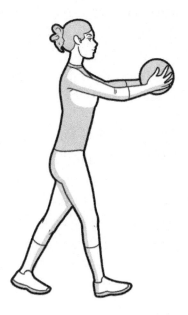

FLOOR EXERCISES

The floor exercises outlined in this guide target various muscle groups that are often overlooked. These movements are carefully selected to cater to the distinct needs of seniors across different ability levels. They will challenge you in different ways to the exercises we have seen so far.

There may appear to be some overlap between floor and core exercises, primarily because many floor exercises also engage the core muscles. However, the main distinction lies in the focus of floor exercises, which is primarily on mobility and stretching. When we have included an exercise in 'floor' when it seems like it should have been included in 'core, it's because of its added advantages, such as better coordination, increased mobility, or the strengthening of specific muscles, including the glutes or posterior chain.

Incorporating these exercises into your routine can improve mobility and enhance your quality of life. Stronger, more flexible people are less prone to accidents, and regular physical activity contributes significantly to an active, independent lifestyle.

Remember, modifications are not a setback but a tool to ensure you can safely and effectively perform the exercises. Progress may be gradual, and patience is essential. Setting realistic goals and celebrating small achievements can make the journey more rewarding and encourage long-term commitment to staying active.

Pelvic Tilt

While it looks simple, the pelvic tilt is an exercise that can be difficult to master. Record yourself doing it and then compare it to the video demonstration to get its true benefit.

It is an introductory exercise beneficial for strengthening your abdominal muscles, enhancing stability when standing, and helping alleviate lower back pain. It's safe for most people and doable for beginners.

Lie on the floor with your knees bent, feet flat, arms extended beside you, and palms facing down. Keep your head, neck, and spine aligned with a natural curve in your lower back, leaving enough space to slide a hand beneath it. Inhale, and as you exhale, engage your abdominal muscles to tilt your tailbone upward, closing the space under your lower back. Feel a gentle stretch in your lower back. Inhale again to return your spine and pelvis to the starting position.

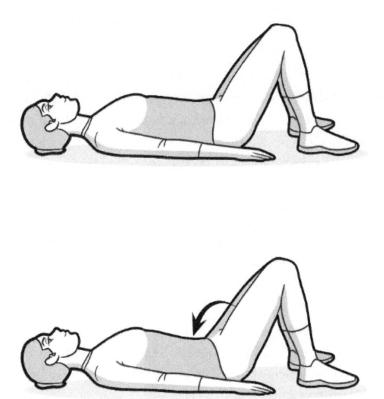

Knee-to-Chest Stretch

The knee-to-chest stretch improves flexibility and mobility in the lower back and hips, alleviating back tension and enhancing muscle circulation. Ideal for starting a flexibility routine, it's a low-impact, safe exercise suitable for most people, including beginners and those with limited mobility.

For this stretch, begin by lying flat on your back, preferably on an exercise mat. Ensure your hips are level and your lower back is in a comfortable, natural position pressed against the floor. With a focus on engaging your core, gently draw one knee toward your chest, holding it with both hands. Take a deep breath, and as you exhale, embrace the stretch, aiming to hold for about 10 seconds. Carefully extend the leg back down to the starting position and switch to the other leg to complete the rep, ensuring you maintain a smooth and controlled movement.

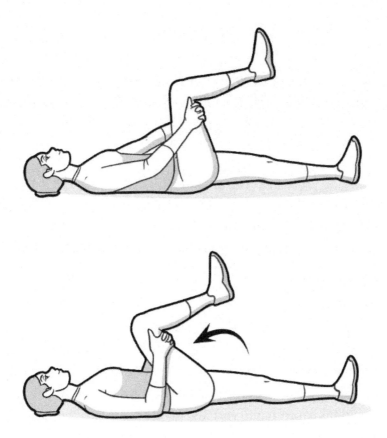

Cat-Cow

The cat-cow stretch is a gentle flow between two yoga poses that warms the body and adds flexibility to the spine. It works the back, torso, and neck and softly stimulates and strengthens the abdominal muscles. It aids in balance by improving spinal mobility, which is crucial for good posture and alignment.

To perform the cat-cow stretch, you'll begin on an exercise mat in a tabletop position, aligning your knees under your hips and your wrists under your shoulders. Aim for a neutral, flat-back position.

Begin to arch your back as you inhale deeply, letting your belly drop toward the floor while lifting your head and tailbone toward the ceiling—this is the 'cow' position. While exhaling, round your spine up toward the ceiling, tucking your chin to your chest and drawing your tailbone under—this is the 'cat' position. These movements are done in a slow, fluid motion, with the transition between the 'cat' and 'cow' positions coordinated with the breath. This exercise is beginner-friendly.

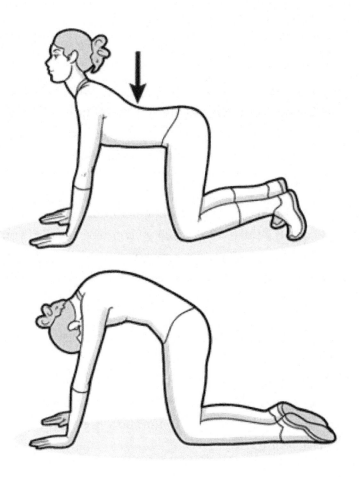

Clamshells

This exercise is designed to bolster hip and glute strength, which is vital in achieving a balanced gait and maintaining proper posture. Regular practice of this movement can enhance your ability to distribute your weight evenly and maintain stability as you walk or stand.

Typically ranked from beginner to intermediate difficulty, the clamshell can be adjusted to match your fitness level. If you find the movement challenging, minimizing the range of motion can make it more manageable. Conversely, incorporating a resistance band around your knees can increase the intensity.

For comfort and support, perform this exercise on a mat. Lie on your side with your knees bent, stacking your legs. Focus on engaging your core as you keep your feet together and lift your top knee, resembling a clamshell opening. Aim to hold this raised position for 2 seconds before gently returning to the start. Repeat the same number of reps on each side.

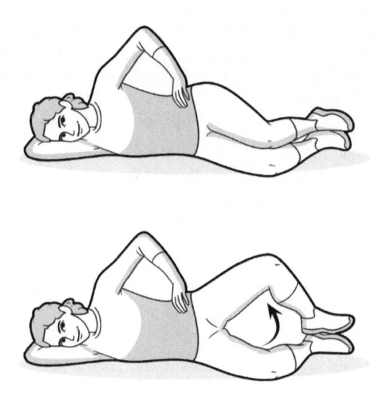

Side-Lying Hip Abduction

The side-lying hip abduction effectively targets the glute medius and the outer thigh muscles. By training the ability to lift the leg sideways away from the body, this exercise enhances stability, particularly when standing on one leg. If not regularly exercised, these muscles can weaken, potentially causing pain, discomfort, and stability problems. This exercise is considered to be at an intermediate level.

To perform, lie on an exercise mat for comfort, on your side with your legs straight. Place the arm closest to the ground under your head for support, letting your head rest fully on your arm, and use your other arm in front for balance. Engage your core, and then slowly lift your upper leg as high as comfortably possible while exhaling. Hold this position briefly for a few seconds before gently lowering your leg. If your body starts to lose alignment, you've likely lifted too high; in this case, decrease your range of motion. Be sure to complete an equal number of reps with each leg.

Beginners should start with a smaller range of motion, lifting the leg just a few inches at first and then gradually increasing the lift beyond the hip level as confidence improves. It's important to avoid raising the leg too quickly; instead, focus on moving it in a controlled, steady manner.

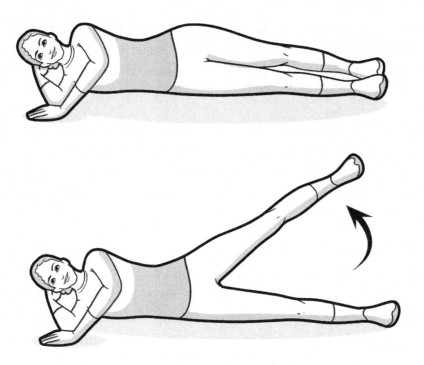

Glute Bridge

The glute bridge is a targeted exercise to enhance core and lower body strength, particularly the gluteal muscles, which are essential for stable movement and reducing back discomfort. By strengthening these areas, you can support better posture and improve lower body function.

This exercise falls into the intermediate category but can be adjusted in intensity. Beginners can start by lifting their hips to a comfortable height and gradually increasing the height as strength improves. For a more challenging variation, straighten one leg at the peak of the bridge.

To begin, lie flat on your back with knees bent, feet flat on the ground, hip-width apart, arms resting by your sides, palms facing down. Keeping your spine neutral, press through your heels and squeeze your glutes as you raise your hips toward the ceiling. Create a straight line from your shoulders to your knees, and avoid arching the lower back. Aim to hold this raised position for 2 seconds before carefully lowering back down to complete the rep.

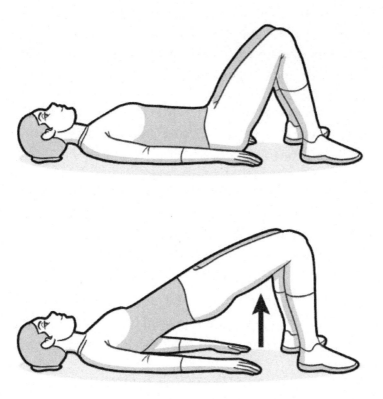

Kneeling to Standing

This is a functional movement that enhances balance, stability, and the smooth transition between positions. It targets the core, back, and legs, providing the strength and support necessary for moving from kneeling to standing with greater ease.

Classed as an intermediate exercise, it can be modified for those who need additional support. Using aids like a chair can provide stability during the transition.

Begin on your knees with a chair positioned beside you for support. Transition into a lunge by placing one foot flat on the ground in front of you, keeping the other knee on the ground. Lean slightly forward, shifting your weight toward your front foot. With one hand on the chair for support, engage your core and leg muscles, and use your front foot to push off the ground, bringing yourself to a standing position. Focus on engaging the glute and hamstring of the leading leg while looking forward and keeping your shoulders pulled back.

Once standing, reverse the motion to return to the initial kneeling position, controlling the descent to avoid any impact on your knees. Complete with both legs leading for one rep.

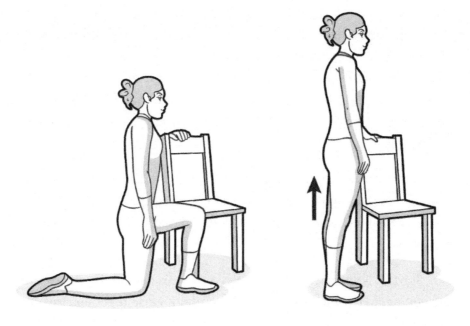

Windshield Wipers

This exercise is a dynamic movement that targets the core and enhances lower back flexibility. It is known for relieving lumbar tension while strengthening the abdominal muscles. This dynamic movement increases the rotational range of motion, indirectly supporting better balance by enhancing core stability and spinal health—key factors in maintaining upright stability during movement.

Labeled as an intermediate-level maneuver, the intensity of this exercise can be adjusted. For a less demanding variation, reduce the range of the knee drops. To increase the difficulty, expand the range of motion.

Start by lying on your back with your knees bent, pointing toward the ceiling, and your feet flat on the ground, close together. Engage your core, then gently tilt your knees to one side until they reach the floor (or as far as you can go.) Return to the center before alternating to the other side. Shift your knees to both sides to complete a rep.

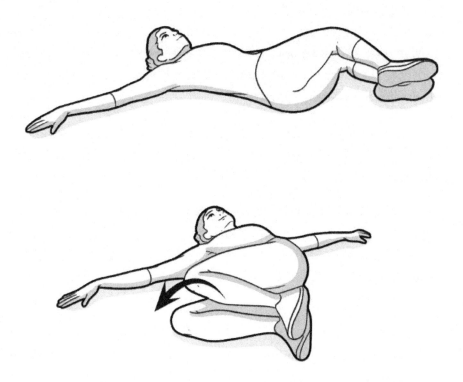

Crawling

Crawling is an exercise that enhances dynamic balance by engaging the core, back, and leg muscles. It promotes stability and fluidity in movements, aiding smooth transitions between positions. As a full-body exercise, it develops motor control and proprioception without placing undue stress on the body.

Categorized as challenging, it's important to note that those with weaker knees or similar concerns should consult a physician before attempting this exercise to ensure it is safe and suitable.

To perform this exercise, begin by positioning yourself on your hands and knees, aligning your knees beneath your hips and wrists beneath your shoulders. Raise your knees a couple of inches off the ground, then move forward by advancing one hand with the opposite knee.

One rep constitutes the movement of your left hand and right foot, then your right hand and left foot. As you gain more confidence and strength, you may gradually increase the distance of your crawl, always emphasizing controlled, stable movements. Maintain a neutral back throughout.

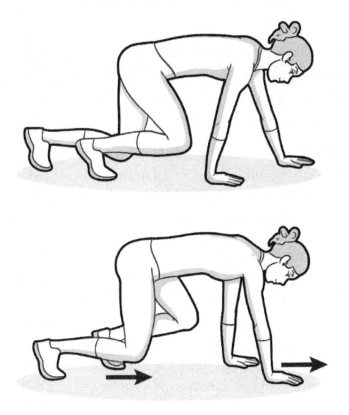

Alternating Superman

The alternating superman effectively engages and fortifies the core, lower back, and gluteal muscles, promoting dynamic balance and flexibility. This exercise is not only pivotal for strengthening but also beneficial for enhancing coordination and stability.

Regarded as a moderately challenging exercise, it offers versatility through modifications. To simplify, you can reduce the elevation of the limbs and the duration of the hold. You can also begin by only doing one leg or arm at a time.

Prepare an exercise mat for comfort. Lie prone with arms extended forward and legs straight. Keep your gaze toward the floor to avoid neck discomfort. Engaging your core and glutes, simultaneously lift one arm and the opposite leg a few inches off the ground, ensuring the lift is manageable and comfortable. Hold this raised position for five seconds before gently returning to the initial pose. Then, alternate to the opposite arm and leg, maintaining a controlled and deliberate movement. Complete on both sides for one rep.

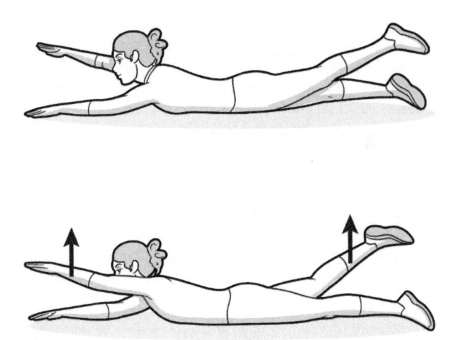

CORE EXERCISES

Core exercises play a crucial role in boosting balance, enhancing strength, and increasing flexibility by targeting the abdominal muscles and their supporting groups. These muscles are fundamental in maintaining proper posture, ensuring stability, and achieving balance, all of which are essential for everyday actions, including standing and bending.

A study by the National Institutes of Health involving seniors aged 65 to 85 engaging in core exercises three times weekly for six weeks demonstrated significant gains in physical capabilities. This underscores the pivotal role core muscles play in our physical functionality.

With aging, our activity often decreases, leading to less use and testing of our core muscles. The core exercises suggested here are specifically designed for seniors, ensuring they are safe and effective while considering their unique needs and any potential limitations. A strong core can remarkably enhance daily activities, from household chores to shopping. It enhances the feeling of having a strong and stable body.

The approach to these exercises should be patient and individualized. Recognize your starting point and progress, advancing to more challenging exercises only when you feel ready. It's vital to practice self-compassion while remaining consistent in your efforts.

This collection of core exercises is curated to cater to seniors, starting with more straightforward exercises that can be modified to suit varying abilities and progressing to more complex ones over time.

Seated Leg Kicks

Seated leg kicks are a dynamic exercise to strengthen the core and engage the lower body, contributing to improved balance and stability. Suitable for a range of abilities from beginner to intermediate, this exercise can be modified to suit individual comfort levels.

To perform seated leg kicks, sit on the edge of a stable chair with your back straight and at about a 30-degree angle. Holding the sides of the chair for stability, extend both legs in front of your body, raising them a few inches off the ground.

Keeping your legs straight and engaging your core, kick your legs in front of you with a moderate range of motion; no need to go above parallel. Ensure your movement is slow and controlled. Hover your back off the backrest very slightly to make the exercise more challenging.

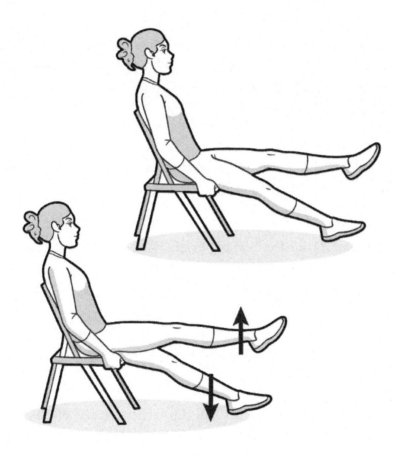

Standing Oblique Crunches

The standing oblique crunch is an effective exercise to specifically target the oblique muscles along the sides of the abdomen. This movement strengthens and promotes flexibility, aiding in proper weight distribution during various actions.

Although a beginner exercise, it requires the simultaneous engagement of the core and coordination of the upper body. You may opt to perform this exercise without weights and gradually introduce light weights to increase intensity.

Stand with your feet planted firmly on the floor, shoulder-width apart. If using a dumbbell, hold it in one hand with your other hand lightly placed behind your head or extended to the side for balance. Engage your core, then bend sideways at the waist, moving toward the hand holding the weight, engaging the obliques. Return to an upright position and switch the weight to the opposite hand, repeating the bend on the other side for a full rep.

You may wish to complete all reps on one side before moving to the other to avoid having to keep switching the weight. Maintain control throughout and perform the movement slowly.

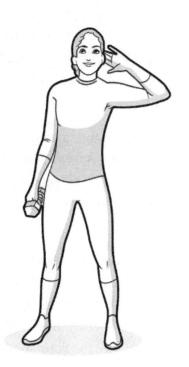
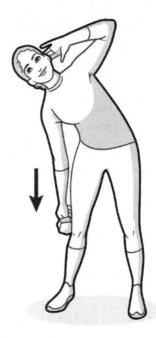

Dead Bug

The dead bug exercise boosts core stability and coordination by engaging multiple limbs. It strengthens the core, indirectly aiding in movements like sitting up and standing, and enhances overall balance. Suitable for various fitness levels, it's a low-impact and effective core workout.

Classified as an intermediate exercise, it can be modified to suit different fitness levels. For those new to the exercise, you can start by moving one arm at a time. Once this is manageable, move on to one leg at a time. Only when you can do these movements with proper form should you move onto the full variation.

First, relax your shoulders and lower back onto the floor, and draw your shoulders away from your ears. Begin with your elbows above your shoulders and palms facing each other. Lift your legs so your knees are above your hips. Then, on an exhale, slowly lower your left arm and right leg until they are a few inches above the floor. Make sure that you keep your lower back pressed against the floor. If you can't, begin with only one arm or leg. Inhale and return to the starting position. Then, repeat on the opposite side for one complete rep.

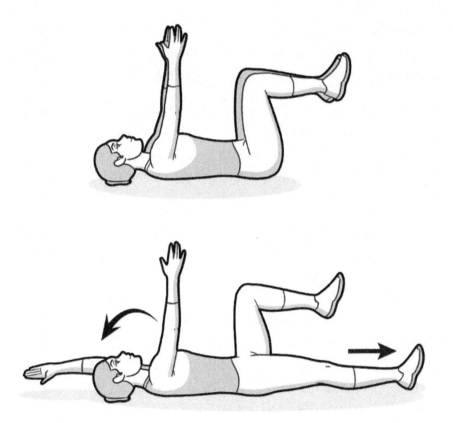

Kneeling Forward Plank

This modified plank variation enhances core strength and stability, offering a less intensive alternative to the full plank. It's particularly suitable for those who find standard planks challenging.

This exercise not only strengthens the abdominal and lower back muscles but also reinforces the pelvic floor, which is crucial for controlling basic body movements. Additionally, by strengthening the core, it indirectly contributes to improved static balance. It is categorized as an intermediate exercise.

To perform this exercise, begin by kneeling on all fours. Transition your weight onto your forearms, aligning elbows under your shoulders, and maintain a straight line from your head to your knees. Ensure your knees remain on the floor, reducing pressure on your back and core. Your toes should rest gently on the ground. Maintain this position for 5-10 seconds, focusing on keeping your core engaged and your body in proper alignment, then relax back to the starting position. Only hold the position as long as you can contract your abdominal muscles and not let your back arch. Do not sink into your shoulders, as this will cause discomfort. Avoid this by pressing your body away from your shoulders toward the ceiling.

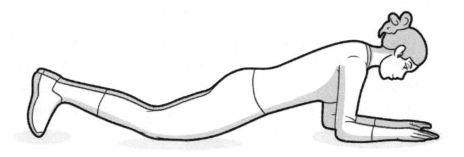

3-Point Stance

The 3-point stance enhances balance by requiring the body to maintain stability while alternating contact points with the ground. It targets core and limb coordination, promoting strength through the engaged muscles. This dynamic exercise challenges you to stabilize using different limbs, which can improve proprioception.

Classified as intermediate, this exercise adds a layer of complexity by challenging your balance through movement. If an exercise mat is too firm and lacks sufficient support, using a bed as an alternative can offer more cushioning. However, it will decrease stability during the exercise.

Position yourself on your hands and knees, aligning your knees under your hips and wrists under your shoulders, maintaining a flat back. Engage your core, glutes, and legs as you lift one leg, extending it directly behind you. Keep the lifted leg in line with your body. Your back must remain flat, not arching either way, throughout. Hold this position for five seconds, ensuring stable, controlled breathing. Then, gently lower your leg back to the starting point and switch to the other leg to complete the rep.

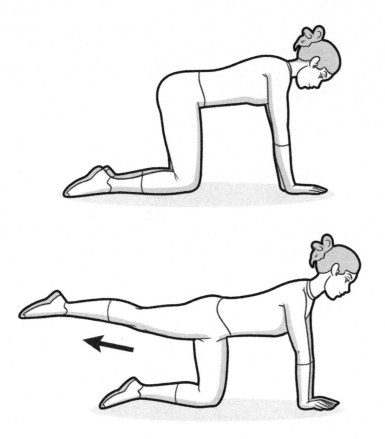

2-Point Stance (Bird Dog)

The 2-point stance is a more challenging variation of the 3-point stance. Again, it is a dynamic exercise that targets core strengthening and promotes stability across the back and legs. This exercise is critical for developing better control over body movements and improving balance and stability.

Categorized as challenging, the 2-point stance tests coordination by requiring independent limb movement. If you find the simultaneous arm and leg extension difficult, stick with the 3-point stance.

Start on your hands and knees, aligning your wrists directly under your shoulders and your knees under your hips. Focus on keeping your spine neutral and your core engaged throughout the movement. As you inhale, extend one arm forward, reaching out as if to touch something in front of you. Concurrently, stretch the opposite leg straight back, creating a straight line from your fingers to your toes.

Aim to hold this extended position for five seconds, maintaining stability and control. Return to the starting position before switching to the opposite arm and leg to complete a rep. Imagine balancing something on your lower back throughout the movement and trying to not let it fall off.

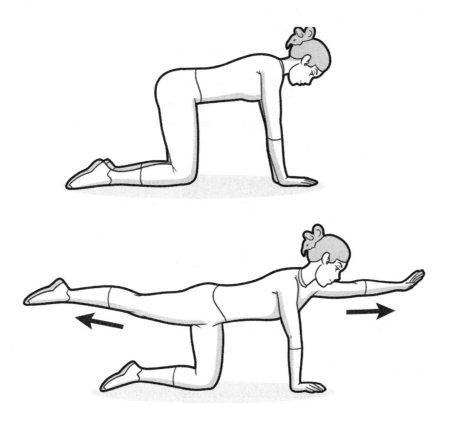

Seated Knee Tucks

The seated knee tuck is a challenging abdominal exercise that also targets the hip flexors and quadriceps, muscles that are integral for controlled movements and stability.

Seated knee tucks can be adjusted to be slightly easier. Beginners may opt to perform the movement with one leg at a time, leaving the other leg extended in front, resting on the ground.

Sit on the floor with your legs extended and hands behind you for support, leaning back at a 45-degree angle. Lift your legs off the ground, then draw your knees toward your chest, contracting your abs without moving your upper body. Squeeze your abs tightly, then slowly return to the starting position. The further behind your hands are, the more support you have and the easier the move will be. Keep your hands on the floor beside your hips for the most challenging variation.

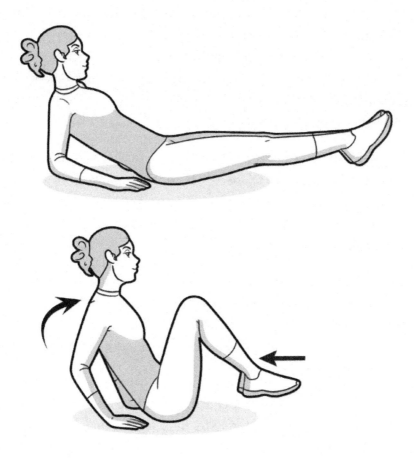

Seated Russian Twist

The seated Russian twist is a highly effective exercise for core strengthening, especially targeting the oblique muscles. It is crucial in enhancing dynamic stability, which is key for maintaining balance during various physical activities and everyday movements. While it engages the lower back muscles, its primary focus is building core rotational strength and stability.

Rated as intermediate, this exercise can be easily adjusted to suit your comfort level. For those new to the movement, limit the rotation to a manageable range that feels comfortable. Consider holding a lightweight object in your hands to add resistance for a greater challenge.

Sit upright on the edge of a chair, with your back very lightly touching the backrest. With your hands clasped in front and your head facing forward, slowly twist your torso to one side as though you're passing over a bag of sugar. Then, smoothly pass it to the other side to complete the rep.

Keep your movements controlled and use your arms to guide the motion, ensuring your core muscles are engaged during the twist. If you are resting your back against the backrest, you won't feel anything, so try to hover slightly. The shallower the angle of your back, the harder it will be.

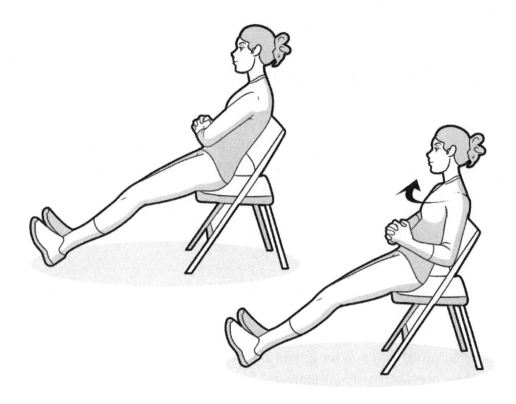

VESTIBULAR EXERCISES

The vestibular system, nestled within the inner ear's vestibular labyrinth, is essential for maintaining equilibrium. It's a crucial yet often undervalued component of our sensory apparatus, directly influencing our capacity to balance and orient ourselves in space. Its health and functionality are paramount for everyday stability and spatial navigation. Research by the National Institutes of Health has underscored its significance, indicating that vestibular rehabilitation can markedly diminish, or even resolve, dizziness and vertigo in most patients.

If you are suffering from dizziness and poor balance, the first thing to do is to speak to a medical professional. They can determine the cause and give you an appropriate treatment plan. If it has been determined that you have issues with your vestibular system, then these exercises can help rehabilitate the damage or difference between the left and right vestibular systems. Go through these exercises with your medical professional to determine the most appropriate for you.

Rehabilitation exercises to enhance this system improve your balance, leading to safer, more controlled movements. They also fortify eye muscles, contributing to stability when our head position changes. They relax the neck and shoulder muscles while training the eye to move independently of the head. They also improve general coordination.

The Brain and Spine Foundation provides comprehensive guidance on vestibular rehabilitation. In the subsequent pages, we will provide instructions on how to perform the exercises safely. Aim to spend 1-2 minutes performing each exercise and only move on to the next group once you are comfortably completing the previous group for three days straight. For example, if you are comfortable doing eye and head movements, only then should you move on to picking up objects and throwing the ball. Once you are comfortable picking up objects and throwing the ball, you can move on to sitting to standing.

All exercises can be performed seated or standing. It's recommended to begin seated and progress to standing only after comfortably mastering all the exercises while seated. Ensure someone is nearby to assist, particularly if there is a risk of falling.

Eye Movement Up-Down

Sit upright in a chair, maintaining a straight back with your head facing forward. Extend your arm straight out in front of you, then slowly raise your arm above your head and down to your waist. As you do, follow your thumb with your eyes while keeping your head still.

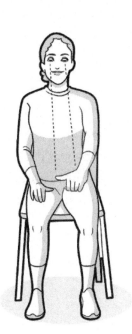
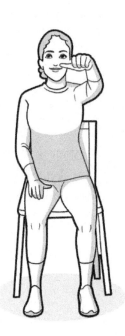
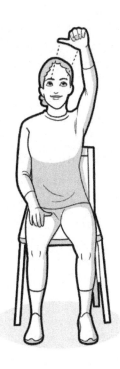

Eye Movement Side-to-Side

Sit with a straight back, facing forward, arm extended out in front of you at eye level. Slowly move your arm to the left, and as you do, follow your thumb with your eye. Keep moving your arm until your thumb is almost out of your peripheral vision. Return your arm to the center and then do the same on the right.

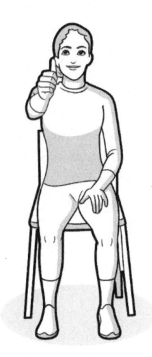
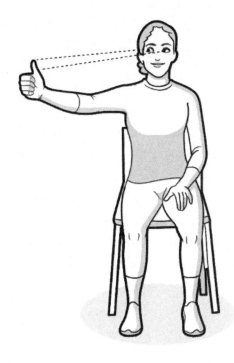

Head Movement Forward-to-Back

Sit upright in a chair or on the edge of a bed. Maintain a straight back and look straight ahead. With your eyes open, gently nod your head forward until your chin nearly touches your chest, then return to the initial position with control. Next, tilt your head backward until you're looking at the ceiling, ensuring the movement is slow and controlled, before returning to the neutral position. Your gaze should follow the movement of your head, with your eyes constantly focusing as your focal point changes.

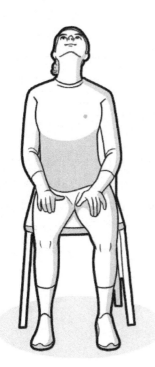
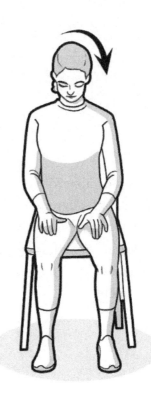

Head Movement Side-to-Side

Sit comfortably with a straight back, keeping your gaze directly ahead to maintain alignment. Turn your head slowly to one side, ensuring the movement is controlled and slow, until you have reached your limit. Return to the central position, then repeat the movement to the opposite side. Keep shifting your focus as your gaze follows your head movements.

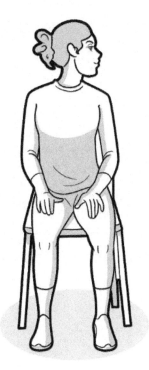
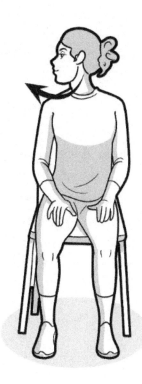

Pick-Up Object in Front

Begin seated with a straight back, eyes forward. Focus on engaging your core as you lean forward smoothly to pick the object off the ground. Grab the object carefully and sit up straight in the chair. Then, return it to the ground with the same level of control and revert to your initial posture. The key is to execute the movement with control and precision to train balance and coordination without risking a fall.

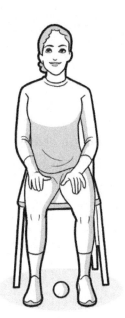
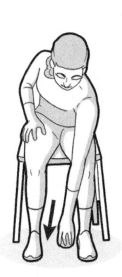
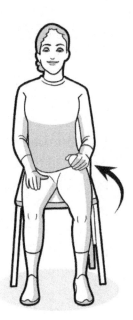

Pick-Up Object Side-to-Side

Position yourself upright in a chair, gaze fixed ahead, with an object like a ball to your side. Keeping your back straight, lean to the side, extending your arm to grab the ball. Pick up the ball smoothly, then place it back down with equal control. After completing the motion on one side, repeat the same number of times on the opposite side to maintain balance in your training.

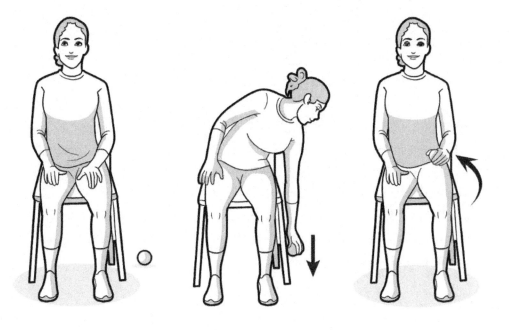

Throwing Ball Hand-to-Hand

To begin, stand with feet planted firmly shoulder-width apart. Hold a ball at eye level and gently toss it from one hand to the other, all while maintaining a forward gaze and minimizing head movement. The aim is to consistently keep the ball at eye level to ensure the eyes track its motion effectively. This exercise not only improves balance and coordination but also sharpens focus. It is best to do this with a tennis ball or something similar.

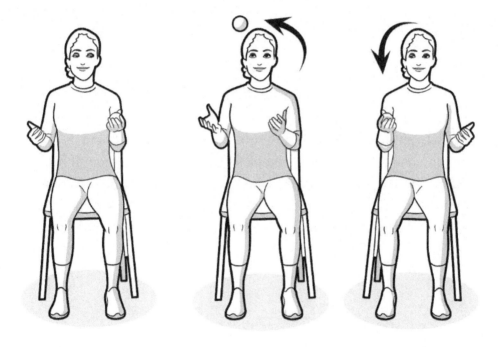

Sitting, Standing, Turning

Begin by sitting on the edge of your bed or a stable chair. Stand up at a measured pace, turn around completely while standing, then sit back down with control. Repeat the movement in the opposite direction, ensuring not to rise or turn too quickly to prevent dizziness. Adjust the speed of the transitions to your comfort level and balance capabilities.

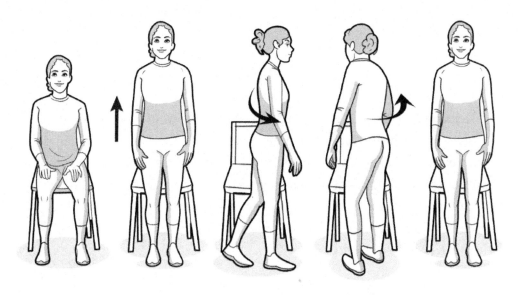

Gaze Stabilization

Focus on an object at eye level 1-3 meters in front of you and slowly turn your head side to side, keeping your eyes on the object. Gradually increase the speed of your head movement as long as the object stays in focus, slowing down if you feel too dizzy. Start the exercise for a duration that causes mild to moderate dizziness, possibly only 10 seconds initially. Gradually increase the time to one minute as you improve and are able to.

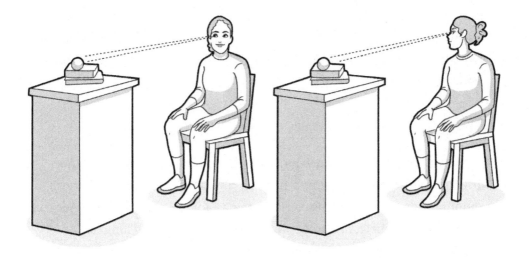

YOUR TWO 30-DAY, 10-MINUTE WORKOUT PLANS

We've developed two daily workout plans and a tracker to integrate easily into any lifestyle. The plans emphasize short, regular workouts over longer, infrequent ones, making it manageable even for those with busy schedules.

What Is in the Plans?

Plan one is for beginners or people who struggle with balance. It comprises mainly beginner and intermediate exercises with more emphasis on seated exercises. Plan two is for people who are more confident, have better balance, and have been practicing longer.

Day one will be a baseline test day, where you'll perform the four balance tests and record your results. The workout schedule will run from Monday through Friday for the next four weeks, with Saturdays and Sundays as designated rest days. On the final day of the plan, you'll have another test day to record your scores, allowing you to compare your progress.

Exercises and Modifications

Each day features a variety of exercises, for example, seated, standing, and core routines, with one vestibular exercise daily. The initial weeks are geared toward easier exercises, gradually progressing to more intermediate and challenging activities in the later weeks. If you're not ready for the challenging exercises by the time you reach them, don't worry; either modify them to make them easier or switch to a beginner/intermediate exercise.

Reps and Sets

Aim for 8-12 reps of each exercise, completing 2 sets. This will take roughly 2 minutes per exercise, including 30-second rest intervals, amounting to a total of 10 minutes of exercise daily. As you grow more confident and comfortable, you can extend your workout time by adding an extra set to each exercise and allowing a bit more rest as needed. However, doing 5 exercises each day is sufficient, so there's no need to add more exercises even if you feel capable.

Tracking Progress

Keep track of your test scores, reps, and any modifications in the tracker below. This record-keeping will be helpful when repeating exercises, as it provides a reference to what you accomplished in previous sessions.

Nutrition and Recovery

Ensure you're eating enough of the right foods to energize you for your workouts. Consuming a small amount of quick-release carbohydrates, like a banana, before exercising is an effective way to fuel your session. A light protein snack post-workout, such as a handful of nuts, can assist in recovery. Proper rest is crucial for both physical and mental recovery, so aim for 7 to 8 hours of sleep per night, but also listen to what your body needs. Remember to always include a warm-up and cool-down in your daily workouts.

What if You Miss a Day?

Despite our best efforts, doing a workout routine daily is not always feasible, and that's perfectly fine. If you miss a day, don't be hard on yourself. However, try to avoid skipping more than one day to avoid losing momentum. If you miss a session, pick up where you left off. For instance, if you missed day 4, proceed with day 4's exercises on day 5 to ensure you cover all focus areas.

Beginner Plan

		Week 1	Week 2	Week 3	Week 4
Monday	1	Seated, Shifting Weight Side-to-Side (B)	Seated, Hip Abduction Side Kicks (B)	Seated, Leg Lift (B)	Seated, Leaning Down on Elbow (I)
	2	Standing, Weight Shifting Front-to-Back (B)	Walking, Sideways (B)	Standing, Sit to Stand (I)	Walking, Toe (I)
	3	Walking, Sideways (B)	Floor, Glute Bridge (I)	Core, 3-Point Stance (I)	Floor, Pelvic Tilt (B)
	4	Floor, Pelvic Tilt (B)	Floor, Windshield Wipers (I)	Floor, Kneeling to Standing (I)	Core, 3-Point Stance (I)
	5	Vestibular, Eye Movement Up-Down	Vestibular, Pick-Up Object Side-to-Side	Vestibular, Eye Movement Up-Down	Vestibular, Sitting, Standing, Turning

		Week 1	Week 2	Week 3	Week 4
Tuesday	1	Seated, Lateral Trunk Flexion (B)	Seated, Leg Lift (B)	Seated, Reaching Partner Required (I)	Seated, Hip Abduction Side Kicks (B)
	2	Standing, Heel Raises (B)	Standing, Weight Shifting Front-to-Back (B)	Standing, Hip Abduction (I)	Standing, Sit to Stand (I)
	3	Floor, Knee-to-Chest Stretch (B)	Walking, Serpentine (I)	Walking, Sideways (B)	Core, Standing Oblique Crunches (B)
	4	Core, Seated Leg Kicks (B)	Floor, Cat-Cow (B)	Floor, Side-Lying Hip Abduction (I)	Floor, Kneeling to Standing (I)
	5	Vestibular, Eye Movement Side-to-Side	Vestibular, Pick-Up Object Side-to-Side	Vestibular, Eye Movement Side-to-Side	Vestibular, Pick-Up Object Side-to-Side

Wednes-day	1	Seated, Shifting Weight Forward-to-Back (B)	Seated, Reaching Partner Required (I)	Seated, Reach With Clasped Hands (I)	Standing, Hip Abduction (I)
	2	Walking, Heel-to-Toe (B)	Standing, Heel Raises (B)	Standing, Weight Shifting Front-to-Back (B)	Walking, Heel (I)
	3	Floor, Cat-Cow (B)	Walking, Heel (I)	Floor, Pelvic Tilt (B)	Floor, Side-Lying Hip Abduction (I)
	4	Core, Standing Oblique Crunches (B)	Floor, Glute Bridge (I)	Floor, Glute Bridge (I)	Floor, Kneeling to Standing (I)
	5	Vestibular, Head Movement Forward-to-Back	Vestibular, Throwing Ball Hand-to-Hand	Vestibular, Head Movement Forward-to-Back	Vestibular, Throwing Ball Hand-to-Hand

Thursday	1	Seated, Trunk Circles (B)	Seated, Shifting Weight Forward-to-Back (B)	Seated, Shifting Weight Side-to-Side (B)	Seated, Reach With Clasped Hands (I)
	2	Standing, Sit to Stand (I)	Standing, Kickback Hip Extension (I)	Standing, Heel Raises (B)	Walking, Heel-to-Toe (B)
	3	Walking, Heel (I)	Walking, Serpentine (I)	Walking, Serpentine (I)	Floor, Cat-Cow (B)
	4	Floor, Clamshells (B)	Floor, Knee-to-Chest Stretch (B)	Floor, Windshield Wipers (I)	Core, 3-Point Stance (I)
	5	Vestibular, Head Movement Side-to-Side	Vestibular, Sitting, Standing, Turning	Vestibular, Head Movement Side-to-Side	Vestibular, Sitting, Standing, Turning

Friday	1	Seated, Leaning Down on Elbow (I)	Seated, Lateral Trunk Flexion (B)	Seated, Trunk Circles (B)	Seated, Hip Abduction Side Kicks (B)
	2	Walking, Heel-to-Toe (B)	Standing, Hip Abduction (I)	Standing, Kickback Hip Extension (I)	Standing, Kickback Hip Extension (I)
	3	Floor, Side-Lying Hip Abduction (I)	Walking, Toe (I)	Floor, Clamshells (B)	Walking, Toe (I)
	4	Core, Standing Oblique Crunches (B)	Floor, Windshield Wipers (I)	Core, Seated Leg Kicks (B)	Core, Seated Leg Kicks (B)
	5	Vestibular, Pick-Up Object in Front	Vestibular, Gaze Stabilization	Vestibular, Pick-Up Object in Front	Vestibular, Gaze Stabilization

Saturday		Rest	Rest	Rest	Rest
Sunday		Rest	Rest	Rest	Rest

Challenging Plan

		Week 1	Week 2	Week 3	Week 4
Monday	1	Standing, Heel Raises (B)	Standing, Hip Abduction (I)	Standing, Bicep Curls for Balance (C)	Standing, Lunge (C)
	2	Walking, Heel-to-Toe (B)	Walking, Heel (I)	Walking, Head Turning (I)	Walking, Grapevine (C)
	3	Floor, Pelvic Tilt (B)	Standing, One-Leg Stand (C)	Floor, Pelvic Tilt (B)	Floor, Side-Lying Hip Abduction (I)
	4	Core, Dead Bug (I)	Floor, Glute Bridge (I)	Core, Standing Oblique Crunches (B)	Floor, Alternating Superman (C)
	5	Vestibular, Pick-Up Object in Front	Vestibular, Pick-Up Object Side-to-Side	Vestibular, Pick-Up Object in Front	Vestibular, Pick-Up Object Side-to-Side

		Week 1	Week 2	Week 3	Week 4
Tuesday	1	Standing, Hip Abduction (I)	Standing, Lunge (C)	Standing, Kickback Hip Extension (I)	Standing, Lateral Lunge (C)
	2	Walking, Heel (I)	Walking, Toe (I)	Walking, Serpentine (I)	Walking, Ball Toss (C)
	3	Floor, Knee-to-Chest Stretch (B)	Floor, Kneeling to Standing (I)	Floor, Knee-to-Chest Stretch (B)	Floor, Crawling (C)
	4	Core, Seated Leg Kicks (B)	Core, 2-Point Stance (Bird Dog) (C)	Core, Seated Knee Tucks (C)	Core, 2-Point Stance (Bird Dog) (C)
	5	Vestibular, Throwing Ball Hand-to-Hand	Vestibular, Sitting, Standing, Turning	Vestibular, Throwing Ball Hand-to-Hand	Vestibular, Sitting, Standing, Turning

Wednes-day	1	Standing, Kickback Hip Extension (I)	Standing, Lateral Lunge (C)	Standing, Step-Up (I)	Standing, Standing Knee Lift (C)
	2	Walking, Toe (I)	Walking, Balance (I)	Walking, Serpentine (I)	Walking, Grapevine (C)
	3	Floor, Cat-Cow (B)	Floor, Windshield Wipers (I)	Floor, Cat-Cow (B)	Floor, Glute Bridge (I)
	4	Core, Standing Oblique Crunches (B)	Core, Seated Russian Twists (I)	Core, Kneeling Forward Plank (I)	Core, Dead Bug (I)
	5	Vestibular, Gaze Stabilization	Vestibular, Throwing Ball Hand-to-Hand	Vestibular, Gaze Stabilization	Vestibular, Throwing Ball Hand-to-Hand

Thursday	1	Standing, Step-Up (I)	Standing, Heel Raises (B)	Standing, Sit to Stand (I)	Standing, Squat (C)
	2	Walking, Backward (I)	Floor, Crawling (C)	Walking, Backward (I)	Walking, Head Turning (I)
	3	Floor, Clamshells (B)	Standing, Standing Knee Lift (C)	Floor, Clamshells (B)	Floor, Crawling (C)
	4	Core, Kneeling Forward Plank (I)	Core, 3-Point Stance (I)	Floor, Kneeling to Standing (I)	Core, Seated Knee Tucks (C)
	5	Vestibular, Pick-Up Object in Front	Vestibular, Pick-Up Object Side-to-Side	Vestibular, Pick-Up Object in Front	Vestibular, Pick-Up Object Side-to-Side

Friday	1	Standing, Sit to Stand (I)	Standing, Squat (C)	Standing, One-Leg Stand (C)	Standing, Bicep Curls for Balance (C)
	2	Walking, Balance (I)	Walking, Heel-to-Toe (B)	Walking, Grapevine (C)	Walking, Ball Toss (C)
	3	Floor, Side-Lying Hip Abduction (I)	Floor, Glute Bridge (I)	Floor, Windshield Wipers (I)	Floor, Alternating Superman (C)
	4	Core, 3-Point Stance (I)	Core, Seated Russian Twists (I)	Core, Seated Leg Kicks (B)	Core, 2-Point Stance (Bird Dog) (C)
	5	Vestibular, Sitting, Standing, Turning	Vestibular, Gaze Stabilization	Vestibular, Sitting, Standing, Turning	Vestibular, Gaze Stabilization

Saturday		Rest	Rest	Rest	Rest
Sunday		Rest	Rest	Rest	Rest

Tracker

Category	Exercise	Difficulty	Date	Reps/ Mod	Date	Reps/ Mod	Date	Reps/ Mod
Seated	Shifting Weight Side-to-Side	B						
Seated	Shifting Weight Forward-to-Back	B						
Seated	Trunk Circles	B						
Seated	Lateral Trunk Flexion	B						
Seated	Leaning Down on Elbow	I						
Seated	Leg Lift	B						
Seated	Hip Abduction Side Kicks	B						
Seated	Reach With Clasped Hands	I						
Seated	Reaching Partner Required	I						
Standing	Weight Shifting Front-to-Back	B						
Standing	Heel Raises	B						
Standing	Hip Abduction	I						
Standing	Kickback Hip Extension	I						
Standing	Step-Up	I						
Standing	Sit to Stand	I						
Standing	One-Leg Stand	C						

Standing	Lunge	C						
Standing	Lateral Lunge	C						
Standing	Standing Knee Lift	C						
Standing	Squat	C						
Standing	Bicep Curls for Balance	C						
Walking	Sideways	B						
Walking	Heel-to-Toe	B						
Walking	Heel	I						
Walking	Toe	I						
Walking	Backward	I						
Walking	Balance	I						
Walking	Head Turning	I						
Walking	Serpentine	I						
Walking	Grapevine	C						
Walking	Ball Toss	C						
Floor	Pelvic Tilt	B						
Floor	Knee-to-Chest Stretch	B						
Floor	Cat-Cow	B						
Floor	Clamshells	B						
Floor	Side-Lying Hip Abduction	I						

Floor	Glute Bridge	I						
Floor	Kneeling to Standing	I						
Floor	Windshield Wipers	I						
Floor	Crawling	C						
Floor	Alternating Superman	C						
Core	Seated Leg Kicks	B						
Core	Standing Oblique Crunches	B						
Core	Dead Bug	I						
Core	Kneeling Forward Plank	I						
Core	3-Point Stance	I						
Core	2-Point Stance (Bird Dog)	C						
Core	Seated Knee Tucks	C						
Core	Seated Russian Twists	I						
Vestibular	Eye Movement Up-Down							
Vestibular	Eye Movement Side-to-Side							
Vestibular	Head Movement Forward-to-Back							
Vestibular	Head Movement Side-to-Side							
Vestibular	Pick-Up Object in Front							
Vestibular	Pick-Up Object Side-to-Side							
Vestibular	Throwing Ball Hand-to-Hand							

Vestibular	Sitting, Standing, Turning							
Vestibular	Gaze Stabilization							
Test	Romberg							
Test	5-Time Sit-to-Stand							
Test	Functional Reach							
Test	Timed Up & Go							

Next Steps

Throughout your 30-day journey, take time to acknowledge your progress. Starting this program demonstrates your commitment to maintaining and improving your health. Your dedication to staying fit is commendable, but remember, the end of these 30 days doesn't mean the end of your fitness journey. Continuous exercise is key to maintaining your progress. Many people choose to repeat this 30-day routine monthly. If you would like to download a blank version of the tracker, you can do so by visiting our website.

For those who completed the Beginner Plan, if you found it comfortable and you feel ready, now it is time to move on to the Challenging Plan. For those who completed the Challenging Plan, the work doesn't stop there. Maintain consistency by repeating the plan, or feel free to add in some of the unused exercises for variation. Consider adding more reps or sets per exercise if you want a greater challenge. Regularly practicing balance exercises is essential if you want to see the long-term benefits.

Beginning an exercise routine can be challenging, but consistent practice promises noticeable improvements in strength, flexibility, balance, and control, leading to a reduced risk of falls and injuries. The hope is that by the end of the month, you will have improved your balance and confidence in your daily life. This routine not only promotes physical fitness but also mental well-being, as regular physical activity has been shown to alleviate depression and anxiety and enhance mental clarity.

IN CONCLUSION

As we age, we naturally experience some decline in our physical strength and ability. Without effort to maintain our fitness, we risk falls, injuries, and potentially losing the capability to live independently. Falls are a common cause of loss of independence among seniors. However, aging doesn't have to mean declining quality of life. Even with limited mobility, there are effective ways to enhance balance, strength, flexibility, and control, significantly reducing the risk of falls and maintaining independence.

In this guide, we've compiled a range of balance exercises tailored for seniors. Each exercise includes clear instructions, benefits, and adaptations to suit individual needs. These exercises are designed not only to improve balance and flexibility but also to enhance strength and coordination.

You've already taken a significant step by reaching this point. Unlike many who only contemplate change, you're actively working toward a healthier, more independent life. By engaging in these exercises, you're proactively safeguarding your health and future independence.

We encourage you to use this guide as a tool for a healthier, safer, and more active lifestyle. Start your journey today and embrace the positive changes it brings. And, if this guide has been a valuable part of your journey, we'd greatly appreciate your feedback through a review. Your thoughts can help others to embark on their journey toward better health and independence.

YOUR VIDEO DEMONSTRATION PASSCODE

baldem123

To Access the Demonstrations:

1. Visit our website, PrimeLife-Wellness.com, and click on 'Video Demonstrations.'

2. Enter the passcode above.

Also on Our Website:

1. **PDF Copy of the Workout Tracker:** At the end of this book, you'll find two 30-day workout plans followed by a blank tracker to record your progress. We've also provided a downloadable PDF version of this tracker on our website, allowing you to reuse it as needed.

2. **Email Community Subscription:** Join our email community to get the following benefits sent straight to your inbox:

   - Be part of our advanced review team and get future books

for free.

- Optimizing nutrition for senior fitness success ebook.

- Breathing techniques to enhance your workout's effectiveness ebook.

Find all these resources on our website, PrimeLife-Wellness.com, or scan the QR code below.

Thank you for being part of our community. Continue your journey toward a healthier, more balanced life with these tools at your disposal.

REFERENCES

A Train Education. (n.d.). *6. Comprehensive Balance Assessment | ATrain Education*. Www.atrainceu.com. https://www.atrainceu.com/content/6-comprehensive-balance-assessment

Aging in Place. (2018, November 9). *Top 10 Elderly Balance Exercises to Improve Balance and Coordination | Updated for 2020*. AgingInPlace.org. https://aginginplace.org/top-10-elderly-balance-exercises-to-improve-balance-and-coordination/

All Active. (n.d.). *Balance exercises for older adults Information Guide Your Health and Fitness*. https://allactive.co.uk/wp-content/uploads/2016/04/Balance-exercises-for-older-adults-AllActive-Information-Guide.pdf

Alzheimer's Association. (2023). *Facts and Figures*. Alzheimer's Disease and Dementia; Alzheimer's Association. https://www.alz.org/alzheimers-dementia/facts-figures

Beaumont Health. (n.d.). *Neurology | Balance Disorder Conditions | Beaumont Health*. Www.beaumont.org. https://www.beaumont.org/conditions/balance-disorders

Berg, R. L., & Cassells, J. S. (2015). *Falls in Older Persons: Risk Factors and Prevention*. Nih.gov; National Academies Press (US). https://www.ncbi.nlm.nih.gov/books/NBK235613/

Biswas, C. (2019, March 25). *Stability Exercises- 15 Best Exercises To Improve Balance*. STYLECRAZE. https://www.stylecraze.com/articles/exercises-for-balance/

Bjerk, M., Brovold, T., Skelton, D. A., & Bergland, A. (2018). Associations between health-related quality of life, physical function and fear of falling in older fallers receiving home care. *BMC Geriatrics, 18*(1). https://doi.org/10.1186/s12877-018-0945-6

Brain & Spine Foundation. (2022, June 24). *Vestibular Rehabilitation Exercises | Fact Sheet | Health Information | Brain & Spine Foundation*. Brain & Spine Foundation. https://www.brainandspine.org.uk/health-information/fact-sheets/vestibular-rehabilitation-exercises/

Bumgardner, W. (2020, May 29). *10 Fun Ways to Add Balance Exercises to Your Walks*. Verywell Fit. https://www.verywellfit.com/add-balance-exercises-to-your-walks-4142274

Burke, K. (2018, May 21). *The importance of warming up and cooling down*. College of Health and Human Sciences. https://chhs.source.colostate.edu/the-importance-of-warming-up-and-cooling-down/

Centers for Disease Control and Prevention. (2019a). *How much physical activity do older adults need?* CDC. https://www.cdc.gov/physicalactivity/basics/older_adults/index.htm

Centers for Disease Control and Prevention. (2019b). *Keep on Your Feet*. Centers for Disease Control and Prevention. https://www.cdc.gov/injury/features/older-adult-falls/index.html

Centers for Disease Control and Prevention. (2020a, March 1). *Physical Activity Recommendations By Age Group*. Centers for Disease Control and Prevention. https://www.cdc.gov/physicalactivity/basics/age-chart.html

Centers for Disease Control and Prevention. (2020b, November 23). *Older Adult Falls Data*. Www.cdc.gov. https://www.cdc.gov/falls/data/index.html

Centers for Disease Control and Prevention. (2021, August 6). *Facts about falls*. Www.cdc.gov. https://www.cdc.gov/falls/facts.html

Cronkleton, E. (2019, December 17). *Cooldown Exercises: 16 Ways to Cool Down with Instructions*. Healthline. https://www.healthline.com/health/exercise-fitness/cooldown-exercises

Davidson, K. (2021, December 6). *Wall Pushups: How to Do This Modified Pushup Variation*. Healthline. https://www.healthline.com/health/fitness-exercise/wall-pushups

DPT, M. R. (2023, June 9). *How To Do a Balance Test at Home (And When to Seek Help)*. Physio Ed. https://physioed.com/how-to-do-a-balance-test-at-home-and-when-to-seek-help/

Effects of Falling on Seniors' Mental Health | Prestige Care. (2021, March 24). Prestige Care; Prestige Care. https://www.prestigecare.com/blog/effects-of-falling-on-seniors-mental-health/

Exercise Cooldown for Seniors, Beginners. (n.d.). Www.youtube.com. https://www.youtube.com/watch?v=TUz3CoihuXQ

Findley, D. (2022, August 30). *Warm-Up Exercises for Seniors or Over 50 • [Video and Guide]*. Over Fifty and Fit. https://overfiftyandfit.com/warm-up-exercises-seniors/

Fox, J. (2021, September 8). *7 Ways To Do Oblique Crunches For A Shredded Midsection | Nutritioneering*. Body Building Meal Plan. https://www.bodybuildingmealplan.com/oblique-crunches/

Freytag, C. (n.d.). *How To Do Windshield Wiper Pose*. Get Healthy U | Chris Freytag. https://gethealthyu.com/exercise/windshield-wiper-pose/

Functional Reach Test (FRT). (n.d.). Physiopedia. Retrieved November 22, 2023, from https://www.physio-pedia.com/Functional_Reach_Test_(FRT)?utm_source=physiopedia&utm_medium=related_articles&utm_campaign=ongoing_internal

Hamilton, V. (2022, August 17). *How to Do a Glute Bridge*. WebMD. https://www.webmd.com/fitness-exercise/how-to-do-glute-bridge

Harvard Health Publishing. (2019). *How medications can affect your balance - Harvard Health*. Harvard Health; Harvard Health. https://www.health.harvard.edu/staying-healthy/how-medications-can-affect-your-balance

Health Care Associates & Community Care Givers. (2013, July 17). *10 Environmental Hazards That Cause Older Adults To Fall & How To Avoid Them | Health Care Associates & Community Care Givers*. Health Care Associates & Community Care Givers. https://healthcareassociates.net/top-10-tripping-hazards-for-older-adults/

Health in Aging. (2016). *Basic Facts about Balance Problems | Aging & Health A-Z | American Geriatrics Society | HealthInAging.org*. Healthinaging.org. https://www.healthinaging.org/a-z-topic/balance-problems/basic-facts

Health, R. (2018, March 19). *Why You Need to Warm Up, Stretch and Cool Down*. Healthlines. https://riverview.org/blog/fitness-2/why-you-need-to-warm-up-stretch-and-cool-down/

Healthline. (2020, May 11). *Balance Exercises for Seniors: 11 Moves to Try*. Healthline. https://www.healthline.com/health/exercise-fitness/balance-exercises-for-seniors

Herman, K., Barton, C., Malliaras, P., & Morrissey, D. (2012). The effectiveness of neuromuscular warm-up strategies, that require no additional equipment, for preventing lower limb injuries during sports participation: a systematic review. *BMC Medicine, 10*(1). https://doi.org/10.1186/1741-7015-10-75

Hinge Health. (n.d.). *Seated Side Bend: Tips and Recommended Variations*. Hingehealth. Retrieved November 22, 2023, from https://www.hingehealth.com/resources/articles/seated-side-bend/

Hoffman, H. (2017, July 18). *5 Best Sitting Balance Exercises for Stroke Patients (With Videos) | Saebo*. Saebo. https://www.saebo.com/blog/5-best-sitting-balance-exercises-stroke-patients-videos/

http://www.facebook.com/BetterHealthWhileAging. (2017, March 9). *10 Types of Medication That May Cause Falls in Aging*. Better Health While Aging. https://betterhealthwhileaging.net/preventing-falls-10-types-of-medications-to-review/

Kahle, N., & Tevald, M. A. (2014). Core Muscle Strengthening's Improvement of Balance Performance in Community-Dwelling Older Adults: A Pilot Study. *Journal of Aging and Physical Activity, 22*(1), 65–73. https://doi.org/10.1123/japa.2012-0132

Kane, E. C., & C.D.S. (n.d.). *Safety Hazards In The Home For The Elderly: Tips On Prevention For Seniors*. Senior Safety Advice. https://seniorsafetyadvice.com/safety-hazards-in-the-home-for-the-elderly/

Kang, K.-Y. (2015). Effects of core muscle stability training on the weight distribution and stability of the elderly. *Journal of Physical Therapy Science, 27*(10), 3163–3165. https://doi.org/10.1589/jpts.27.3163

Khanna, R. (2022, June 5). *6 Fun and Effective Ways You Can Include Balance Exercises in Your Walks*. Www.sportskeeda.com. https://www.sportskeeda.com/health-and-fitness/6-balance-exercises-can-include-walks

Konrad, H. R., Girardi, M., & Helfert, R. (1999). Balance and Aging. *The Laryngoscope, 109*(9), 1454–1460. https://doi.org/10.1097/00005537-199909000-00019

Lee, S. (2021). Falls associated with indoor and outdoor environmental hazards among community-dwelling older adults between men and women. *BMC Geriatrics, 21*(1). https://doi.org/10.1186/s12877-021-02499-x

Liu, M., Hou, T., Li, Y., Sun, X., Szanton, S. L., Clemson, L., & Davidson, P. M. (2021). Fear of falling is as important as multiple previous falls in terms of limiting daily activities: a longitudinal study. *BMC Geriatrics, 21*(1). https://doi.org/10.1186/s12877-021-02305-8

Lo'Aids. (2021, April 26). *50 Inspiring Senior Fitness Quotes To Keep You Moving*. Lo'Aids. https://loaids.com/senior-fitness-quotes/

Lopes Da Silva, T., Vieira Da Motta, V., José, W., Ferreira Pinto, P., Santos, P., Parreira, D., & Pereira De Paiva, E. (2021). SUPPLEMENTARY EDITION 2 Rev Bras Enferm. *Rev Bras Enferm, 74*(2), 20200400. https://doi.org/10.1590/0034-7167-2020-0400

Luff, C. (n.d.). *10 Core Strengthening Exercises for Runners*. Verywell Fit. https://www.verywellfit.com/core-strengthening-exercises-for-runners-2911910

M.D, H. L. (2013, October 31). *Balance training seems to prevent falls, injuries in seniors*. Harvard Health Blog. https://www.health.harvard.edu/blog/balance-training-seems-to-prevent-falls-injuries-in-seniors-201310316825

Maharaj, S. (2021, September 6). *Static Balance vs. Dynamic Balance Exercises*. Propel Physiotherapy. https://propelphysiotherapy.com/exercise/static-balance-vs-dynamic-balance-exercises/#:~:text=Static%20balance%20is%20our%20ability

Mancini, M., & Horak, F. B. (2010). The relevance of clinical balance assessment tools to differentiate balance deficits. *European Journal of Physical and Rehabilitation Medicine, 46*(2), 239–248. https://www.ncbi.nlm.nih.gov/pmc/articles/PMC3033730/

Mangar. (2017, May 3). *The Unspoken Emotional Impact Of Falling In Old Age - Mangar US*. Mangarhealth.com. https://mangarhealth.com/us/by-winncare/market-insights/unspoken-emotional-impact-falling-old-age/

Mayo Clinic. (n.d.-a). *Balance exercises: Step-by-step guide*. Mayo Clinic. https://www.mayoclinic.org/healthy-lifestyle/fitness/in-depth/balance-exercises/art-20546836

Mayo Clinic. (n.d.-b). *Weight-training do's and don'ts*. Mayo Clinic. https://www.mayoclinic.org/healthy-lifestyle/fitness/in-depth/weight-training/art-20045842#:~:text=You%20might%20be%20tempted%20to

Mayo Clinic. (2018). *Mild cognitive impairment - Symptoms and causes.* Mayo Clinic. https://www.mayoclinic.org/diseases-conditions/mild-cognitive-impairment/symptoms-causes/syc-20354578

MD, M. J. (2021, October 25). *Standing Up is Still Doing a Little Exercise! • MyHeart*. MyHeart. https://myheart.net/articles/standing-up-is-still-doing-a-little-exercise/

Medical News Today. (2022, July 8). *Balance exercises: Types, benefits, and more.* Www.medicalnewstoday.com. https://www.medicalnewstoday.com/articles/balance-exercises#older-adults

Medications Can Cause Balance Problems. (n.d.). The Arbors Assisted Living Community. https://thearborsassistedliving.com/medications-can-cause-balance-problems/

Medline Plus. (n.d.). *Balance Tests: MedlinePlus Medical Test*. Medlineplus.gov. Retrieved November 22, 2023, from https://medlineplus.gov/lab-tests/balance-tests/#:~:text=Other%20conditions%20can%20also%20cause

Mehegan, L. (2022, October 5). *Walking: Attitudes and Habits of Adults Age 50 and Older*. AARP; AARP. https://www.aarp.org/pri/topics/health/prevention-wellness/walking-attitudes-habits-adults-50-older.html

Melone, L. (n.d.). *7 Dynamic Warm Ups*. Arthritis Foundation. https://www.arthritis.org/health-wellness/healthy-living/physical-activity/other-activities/7-dynamic-warm-ups

Murman, D. (2015). The Impact of Age on Cognition. *Seminars in Hearing*, *36*(03), 111–121. https://doi.org/10.1055/s-0035-1555115

Murphy, M. (2021, June 2). *Off balance? May be a nerve condition.* Mayo Clinic Health System. https://www.mayoclinichealthsystem.org/hometown-health/speaking-of-health/feeling-off-balance-a-nerve-condition-may-be-to-blame

Murray, K. (n.d.). *Balance Exercises for Stroke Patients*. Stroke Rehab. https://www.stroke-rehab.com/balance-exercises.html#gsc.tab=0

National Institute On Aging. (n.d.). *Falls and Fractures in Older Adults: Causes and Prevention*. National Institute on Aging. https://www.nia.nih.gov/health/falls-and-falls-prevention/falls-and-fractures-older-adults-causes-and-prevention

Nebula Physio. (n.d.). *5 Simple Exercises to Improve Balance*. Www.nebula-Physio.co.uk. https://www.nebula-physio.co.uk/advice/exercises-to-improve-balance

NHS. (2017, October 17). Balance exercises. *NHS Choices*. https://www.nhs.uk/live-well/exercise/strength-and-flexibility-exercises/balance-exercises/

NHS Inform. (2020, April 30). *Warm-up and cool-down*. Www.nhsinform.scot. https://www.nhsinform.scot/healthy-living/keeping-active/before-and-after-exercise/warm-up-and-cool-down

Nunez, K. (2019a, July 12). *12 Exercises for Dynamic Flexibility*. Healthline; Healthline Media. https://www.healthline.com/health/exercise-fitness/dynamic-flexibility

Nunez, K. (2019b, August 7). *Are Rest Days Important for Exercise?* Healthline; Healthline Media. https://www.healthline.com/health/exercise-fitness/rest-day

Older Adults and Balance Problems. (n.d.). National Institute on Aging. https://www.nia.nih.gov/health/falls-and-falls-prevention/older-adults-and-balance-problems

Örgün, E. (2020). The effect of static and dynamic core exercises on dynamic balance, spinal stability, and hip mobility in female office workers. *Turkish Journal of Physical Medicine and Rehabilitation*, *66*(3), 271–280. https://doi.org/10.5606/tftrd.2020.4317

Orthopaedic Associates. (2017, November 10). *Common Fall Injuries*. Orthopaedic Associates of Central Maryland. https://www.mdbonedocs.com/common-fall-injuries/

Ortiz, D. (2020, August 5). *7 Causes of Balance Issues in the Golden Years*. Home Care Assistance of Jefferson County. https://www.homecareassistancejeffersonco.com/what-can-be-causing-my-elderly-parents-balance-difficulties/

Paplou, V., Schubert, N., & Pyott, S. (2021, September 3). *Age-Related Changes in the Cochlea and Vestibule: Shared Patterns and Processes*. Frontiers. https://www.frontiersin.org/articles/10.3389/fnins.2021.680856/full

Pardue-Spears, C. (2018, February 5). *Common Problems Faced by the Elderly in the US*. Family Matters. https://familymattershc.com/common-problems-for-elderly/

physiopedia. (2015). *Coordination Exercises*. Physiopedia. https://www.physio-pedia.com/Coordination_Exercises

Physitrack. (n.d.-a). *How to perform the Ankle Pumps - Physitrack*. Www.physitrack.com. https://www.physitrack.com/en-gb/exercise-library/how-to-perform-the-ankle-pumps-exercise

Physitrack. (n.d.-b). *How to perform the Grapevine exercise - Physitrack*. Www.physitrack.com. https://www.physitrack.com/en-gb/exercise-library/how-to-perform-grapevine-exercise

Pizer, A. (2021, December 8). *How to Do Cat-Cow Stretch (Chakravakasana) in Yoga*. Verywell Fit. https://www.verywellfit.com/cat-cow-stretch-chakravakasana-3567178

Premier Neurology. (2021, November 5). *The Vestibular System: What It is and How It Affects Balance*. Premier Neurology & Wellness Center. https://premierneurologycenter.com/blog/the-vestibular-system-what-it-is-and-how-it-affects-balance/#:~:text=The%20vestibular%20system%20is%20a

Prendergast, C. (2022, December 7). *Exercise Warmup for Seniors*. Physio Ed. https://physioed.com/exercise-warmup-for-seniors/

Propel Physiotherapy. (n.d.). *Front Back Weight Shifting - Dynamic Balance*. Www.youtube.com. Retrieved November 22, 2023, from https://www.youtube.com/watch?v=h9N1I3cT070

Pysio Pedia. (n.d.). *Single Knee to Chest Stretch*. Physiopedia. https://www.physio-pedia.com/Single_Knee_to_Chest_Stretch

Rodriguez, J. (2022, December 20). *What are the problems faced by elderly in our society?* Griswold Home Care. https://www.griswoldhomecare.com/blog/2022/december/what-are-the-problems-faced-by-elderly-in-our-so/

Rogers, P. (2022, September 22). *How to Build a Workout for Getting Better Results*. Verywell Fit. https://www.verywellfit.com/beginners-guide-to-sets-repetitions-and-rest-intervals-3498619

Runner's World. (2023, January 30). *How to do the clamshell exercise - and strengthen your hips and glutes*. Runner's World. https://www.runnersworld.com/uk/training/cross-training/a42667936/clamshell-exercise/

Salzman, B. (2010). Gait and Balance Disorders in Older Adults. *American Family Physician, 82*(1), 61–68. https://www.aafp.org/pubs/afp/issues/2010/0701/p61.html

Santos-Longhurst, A. (2019, July 15). *Proprioception: What It Is, Problems, Diagnosis, Treatment & More*. Healthline. https://www.healthline.com/health/body/proprioception

Schrift, D. (n.d.). *From Weak and Wobbly to Strong and Stable*. Eldergym Fitness for Seniors. https://eldergym.com/chair-exercises-for-seniors/

Set, S. F. (n.d.). *Heel Touches: Correct Form, Muscles Worked, & Alternatives*. SET for SET. https://www.setforset.com/blogs/news/heel-touches

Sharma, K. G., & Gupta, A. K. (2020). Efficacy and Comparison of Vestibular Rehabilitation Exercises on Quality of Life in Patients with Vestibular Disorders. *Indian Journal of Otolaryngology and Head & Neck Surgery, 72*(4), 474–479. https://doi.org/10.1007/s12070-020-01920-y

Sherrington, C., Fairhall, N., Wallbank, G., Tiedemann, A., Michaleff, Z. A., Howard, K., Clemson, L., Hopewell, S., & Lamb, S. (2019). Exercise for preventing falls in older people living in the community: An abridged Cochrane systematic review. *British Journal of Sports Medicine, 54(15)*. Retrieved from https://bjsm.bmj.com/content/54/15/885.info

Shoair, O. A., Nyandege, A. N., & Slattum, P. W. (2011). Medication-Related Dizziness in the Older Adult. *Otolaryngologic Clinics of North America, 44*(2), 455–471. https://doi.org/10.1016/j.otc.2011.01.014

Spotebi. (2015, May 2). *Seated Knee Tucks | Illustrated Exercise Guide*. SPOTEBI. https://www.spotebi.com/exercise-guide/seated-knee-tucks/

Stefanacci, R., & Wilkinson, J. (n.d.). *Falls in Older Adults - Geriatrics*. Merck Manuals Professional Edition. Retrieved November 22, 2023, from https://www.merckmanuals.com/professional/geriatrics/falls-in-older-adults/falls-in-older-adults?autoredirectid=22738

Steinhilber, B. (2018, November 28). *Stretching is more than a cool down. Here's why you should consider it exercise*. NBC News; NBC News. https://www.nbcnews.

com/better/health/stretching-more-cool-down-here-s-why-you-should-consider-ncna901371

Talarska, D., Strugała, M., Szewczyczak, M., Tobis, S., Michalak, M., Wróblewska, I., & Wieczorowska – Tobis, K. (2017). Is independence of older adults safe considering the risk of falls? *BMC Geriatrics*, *17*(1). https://doi.org/10.1186/s12877-017-0461-0

The Three Components of Balance | Macht Medical Group. (n.d.). Macht Medical Group. http://www.machtmedicalgroup.com/2015/03/see-no-evil-hear-no-evil-feel-no-evil/

Theresa. (2020, September 30). *Fall hazards for seniors at home | Elderly Fall Prevention*. Elderly Fall Prevention. https://elderlyfallprevention.com/fall-hazards-for-seniors-at-home

Three Spires Physical Therapy. (n.d.). *ThreeSpires Physiotherapy*. Www. threespiresphysiotherapy.co.uk. https://www.threespiresphysiotherapy.co.uk/news-articles/the-5-best-balance-exercises/

Timed Up and Go Test (TUG). (n.d.). Physiopedia. Retrieved November 22, 2023, from https://www.physio-pedia.com/Timed_Up_and_Go_Test_(TUG)?utm_source=physiopedia&utm_medium=related_articles&utm_campaign=ongoing_internal

Tran, A. (2020, June 3). *Balance Exercises for Stroke Patients: How to Improve Stability*. Flint Rehab. https://www.flintrehab.com/balance-exercises-for-stroke-patients/

Very Well Health. (n.d.). *Pelvic Tilt Exercise for People With Back Pain*. Verywell Health. https://www.verywellhealth.com/pelvic-tilt-exercise-for-your-lower-back-296802

Vyazovskiy, V. (2015). Sleep, recovery, and metaregulation: explaining the benefits of sleep. *Nature and Science of Sleep*, *7*(7), 171. https://doi.org/10.2147/nss.s54036

Yorkville Sportsmed. (n.d.). *The Dead Bug Exercise And How You Can Do It Perfectly*. Physiotherapists in Toronto | Yorkville Sports Medicine Clinic. https://www.yorkvillesportsmed.com/blog/the-dead-bug-exercise-and-how-you-can-do-it-perfectly

Zhang, R., Liu, B., Bi, J., & Chen, Y. (2020). Relationship Between Chronic Conditions and Balance Disorders in Outpatients with Dizziness: A Hospital-Based Cross-Sectional Study. *Medical Science Monitor*, *27*. https://doi.org/10.12659/msm.928719